Nail The Diagnosis

What Our Fingernails Reveal About Our Health and Illness

Mark E. Williams, M.D.

Copyright © 2017 Mark E. Williams, M.D.

All rights reserved.

ISBN-13: 9781520634586

DEDICATION

To my wife, Jane

And our sons, John and James

With gratitude for the past,

Loving service for the present,

And responsibility for the future.

NAIL THE DIAGNOSIS:

WHAT OUR FINGERNAILS TELL US ABOUT HEALTH AND ILLNESS

CONTENTS

Preface And Acknowledgments

1. Basic Information

2. Observations Of The Lunula

3. Abnormalities Of Nail Shape

4. Abnormalities Of The Nail Surface

5. Separation Of The Nail From The Nail Bed (Onycholysis)

6. Focal Discolorations Of The Nail

7. Generalized Nail Discoloration

8. Abnormalities Around The Nail

9. Case Presentations

10. Answers To Case Presentations

Bibliography

Mark E. Williams, M.D.

PREFACE AND ACKNOWLEDGMENTS

"It's not what you look at that matters, it's what you see."

—Henry David Thoreau

"**Discipline is the bridge between goals and accomplishment.**"

— Jim Rohn

The goal of this book is to assist the curious, motivated clinician in becoming a more perceptive observer of fingernails to improve one's skills in bedside diagnostic examination. Achieving this goal will depend on the clarity of presentation in this book and on the learner's patience, self-discipline, honesty, and restraint in studying and practicing the appropriate skills.

Medical observation is an active, creative process, part of what we already do in the midst of our daily activities. It is highly portable and efficient and is useful in other areas of our personal growth and conscious evolution. The intention of medical observation is to appreciate the truth in the light of the moment, the reality behind the appearance.

The fingernail assessment is an essential part of the physical examination. This approach is especially satisfying when it promptly leads to an accurate diagnosis and to the patient's relief of suffering and distress. It is difficult to overstate the potential utility of this information that is hidden in plain view. Exemplary technique when associated with a caring manner immediately reflects the clinician's competence to the patient and family members.

Physical diagnosis skills, a core aspect of clinical care, are declining, perhaps on the mistaken notion that advanced technology can replace skillful bedside diagnostic examination. Extremely valuable clinical information can be detected from the fingernails and sadly most modern practitioners neglect much of this readily available observational evidence. Every day, numerous people undergo technological procedures for human predicaments that could have been identified by a careful history and thoughtful physical examination more rapidly and efficiently and at less expense and inconvenience. My book, *Geriatric*

Physical Diagnosis: A Guide to Observation and Assessment, published by McFarland & Company, Inc. attempts to bridge the growing chasm between motivated learners and expert clinical skill.

Do we really need a handbook of fingernail observations? Dermatologists or hand surgeons are the main authors of other books on fingernails. This manual is not meant to be an exhaustive compendium. Diagnostic utility and useful observations have been favored over interesting, but useless minutia. The approach is unapologetically personal and shows one person's way to systematically examine and interpret fingernail findings. It is what I use in my daily clinical practice and is not meant to be a comprehensive evidence based review of digital dermatology.

This book does not address fingernail observations used for forensic purposes. Numerous studies show how fingernail clippings can be analyzed for DNA, heavy metals and a variety of other substances including drug and alcohol metabolites. This burgeoning area is far beyond the scope of this monograph. Likewise I have emphasized acquired findings, especially clues to underlying illness over congenital abnormalities. I have also omitted fingernail observations that require additional equipment such as a dissecting microscope, ultrasound or radiographs.

My secondary intention is to make the material available to a general audience. Healthcare is changing and the more we know about our own health the more effective we can be in making wise decisions when we interact with healthcare professionals.

Fundamental observations refined and prospectively validated through over thirty-five years of active, hands on, clinical practice forms the basis of the work. However, I claim no originality for the interpretations, as my experience is the product of a vast variety of sources: instructors and mentors, current and past textbooks, journal articles and periodicals, discussions with students and colleagues, and of course interactions with my patients and their families. It will not surprise me if others do not uniformly share my clinical impressions. After all, there are many ways to interpret observations and professionals should be expected to sometimes disagree. But the more complete our understanding of subtle fingernail findings in physical diagnosis the better prepared we will be to work with our patients to keep them smiling and happy for as long as possible.

I owe a special thanks to numerous medical students and medical residents for encouraging me to share these observations into a useable monograph. Drs. Kenneth Greer, James McCabe, Kenneth Kotz, and Billy McNulty deserve special mention for sharing some images from their active practices. Finally, I sincerely thank each of my patients who enthusiastically agreed to let me photograph their nails so that we could learn from their circumstances.

Chapter 1

Basic Information

GETTING STARTED

Each of us carries the last six months of our medical record on the approximately ten square centimeters of keratin comprising the fingernails. Our nails are an essential part of our fingers and toes providing protection, temperature regulation, and tactile sensation. A wealth of useful information is available: the manicure can reveal state of health, nutritional status, past events, personality, occupation and one's inner state (See Table 1).

Table 1. Information available from Observing Fingernails

Overall vitality	Nutritional status
Inner emotional state	Cardiovascular function
Cerebral dominance	Possible malignancy
Occupations and hobbies	Liver disease
Six months of past medical history	Kidney disease
Toxic exposures	Endocrine disorders
Rheumatic conditions	Dermatological concerns

HOW TO IDENTIFY SYSTEMIC ILLNESS

Systemic illness generally shows nail changes on all or most of the nails, while local conditions affect only one or two nails. Often the toenails are also involved in systemic illness. The thumb may reveal more extensive nail changes given its increased size and can serve as a point of verification when systemic illness is inferred from noting changes on other nails (since most systemic illnesses affecting the nails should be visible on the thumb nail).

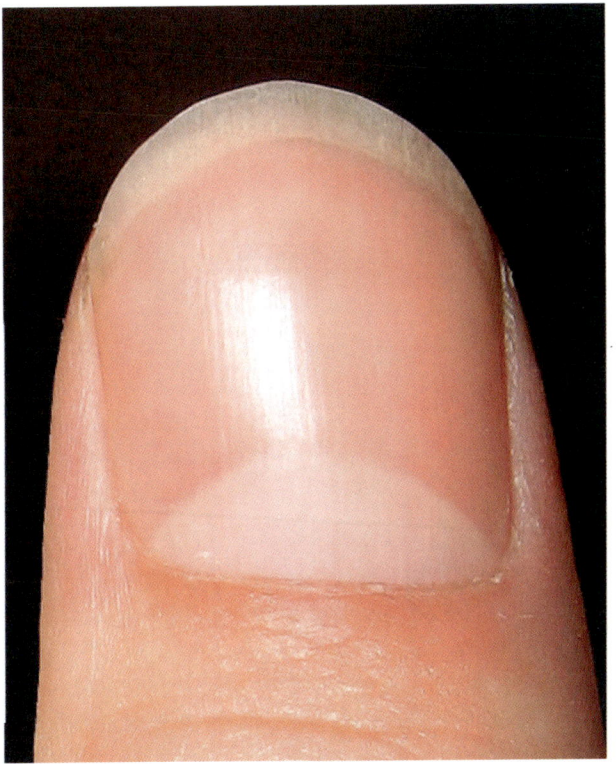

Normal Fingernail

FINGERNAIL ANATOMY

The nail plate is the nail itself is composed of specialized keratin that is similar to the hooves of animals. The nail structure allows a number of complex activities such as picking up small objects and facilitates tactile sensation by providing a firm background. In addition to protecting the fingertip, the nails can be used as tools such as pincers or weapons.

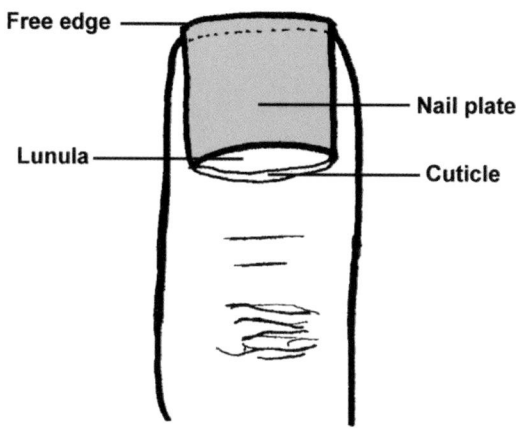

Normal Fingernail

The basic parts of the nail are the nail plate, the cuticle, the lunula, and the free edge (the part we clip when it gets too long).

The nail is composed of approximately 25 layers of dead compressed keratinized cells usually a quarter to a half of a millimeter thick. The cells have specialized desmosomes, intracellular linkages and adhesives to form a tight bond across the nail. In cross section the nail has 3 layers. The most superficial layer is hardened keratin with overlapping cells that produce a shiny, smooth surface. The middle layer is the softest and thickest and has keratin fibers oriented perpendicular to the axis of nail growth. Disulfide bonds from sulfur containing amino acids (primarily cysteine) form an adhesive. The deepest layer of the nail basically binds the nail plate to the nail bed.

NAIL GROWTH

Nail growth is continuous. It takes about six months for a fingernail in an elderly person to completely grow out. Cold temperature can slow growth rates but not to any clinically significant degree. There are no gender differences in growth rate. Toenails take approximately 12 months to grow out fully.

The middle finger nail grows the fastest followed by the

forefinger and ring finger. The little finger has the slowest growth rate. Aging slows the growth rate from approximately three months in childhood to the six months in 70 year olds. Nails in elderly people are also thicker than in younger people. Thin nails in a post- menopausal woman raise the possibility of metabolic bone disease. The nails of the dominant hand grow slightly quicker than the non-dominant nails, probably because minor trauma accelerates nail growth. Conversely, immobility slows the growth rate of fingernails. Dietary factors may affect nail growth but the scientific evidence is not conclusive. Biotin appears to strengthen fingernails.

Poisoning from Bajiaolian (Dysosma pleianthum), used in Chinese herbal medicine for a variety of conditions can cause severe toxicity including complete cessation of nail growth.

Understanding the growth rate is very useful because the time interval from a critical event can be estimated from the location of a nail lesion. For example, a white line appearing transversely halfway up the nail suggests an acute illness producing the line occurred three months earlier. Regular observation will demonstrate its timely progression to the end of the nail edge.

THE NORMAL SEQUENCE OF THE EXAMINATION

The key to examining the fingernails is to appreciate what is normal (or a normal variation) and what is not normal. Some signs of illness are very subtle and paying attention to small details and having a systematic pattern to your observations helps to avoid overlooking something potentially useful.

It is critical to examine the nails in adequate light. Gently rotate the nail in the light so that the reflection highlights all aspects of the nail.

The basic sequence of the examination is listed below:

1- Initial impressions

2- Inspect the lunula

3- Observe the nail shape and nail surface

4- Appreciate any changes in the nail color

5- Examine the tissue around the nails (paronychium)

6- Compare hands (to appreciate symmetry and distribution of findings)

7- Note skin and joint conditions

In the interest of full disclosure I do not always follow this sequence. What usually enters my awareness is an appreciation of an abnormality or constellation of anomalies. Nonetheless this sequence is helpful as an organized way to share fingernail observations and perceptions.

    Our fundamental intention is to appreciate the truth in the light of the moment (the reality behind the appearance) and any fingernail clues are basically mosaics in the overall pattern of illness.

NAIL POLISH

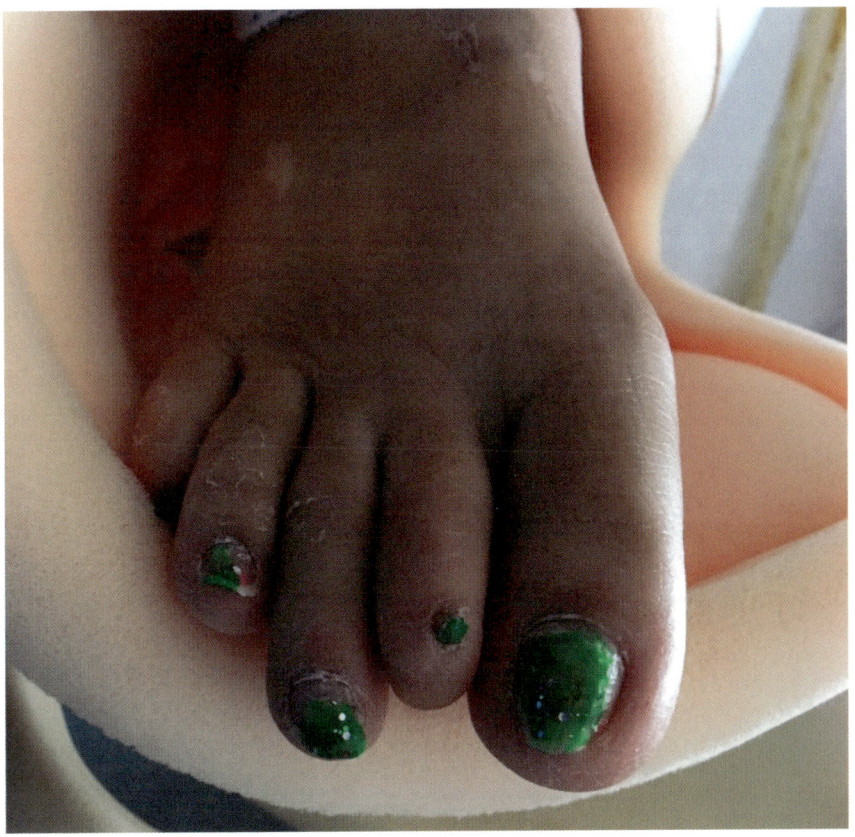

Green nail polish for St. Patrick's Day

Distance from base and line of polish gives approximate date of application (nails grow approximately 0.1mm/ day). The date of the manicure suggests when the person last felt reasonably well. So seeing a recent application in an ill person could reflect an acute process or exacerbation while a more distant manicure suggests significant chronic illness or a change in fortune. Picking at the polish reflects nervousness and agitation. Toenail polish suggests unusual flexibility, a friendly helper or someone who enjoys pedicures. Chronic exposure to nail polish can produce a toxic chemical contact especially to triphenyl phosphate. Nail polish may affect pulse oximetry readings in the acute care setting. The image shows green toenail polish in a middle-aged woman who presented to the hospital in a coma. The amount of nail growth corresponded with the timing for St. Patrick's Day for the application of the nail polish and it was a useful clue to end stage liver disease secondary to alcohol use.

Chapter 2

Observations of the Lunula

EXAMINING THE LUNULA

Notice the lunula, the pale crescent moon-like coloration at the base of the nail. It represents the leading edge of the nail matrix where the nail is produced. No clinical condition causes the lunula to grow in size although it can be large in congenital cyanotic heart disease such as pulmonary stenosis.

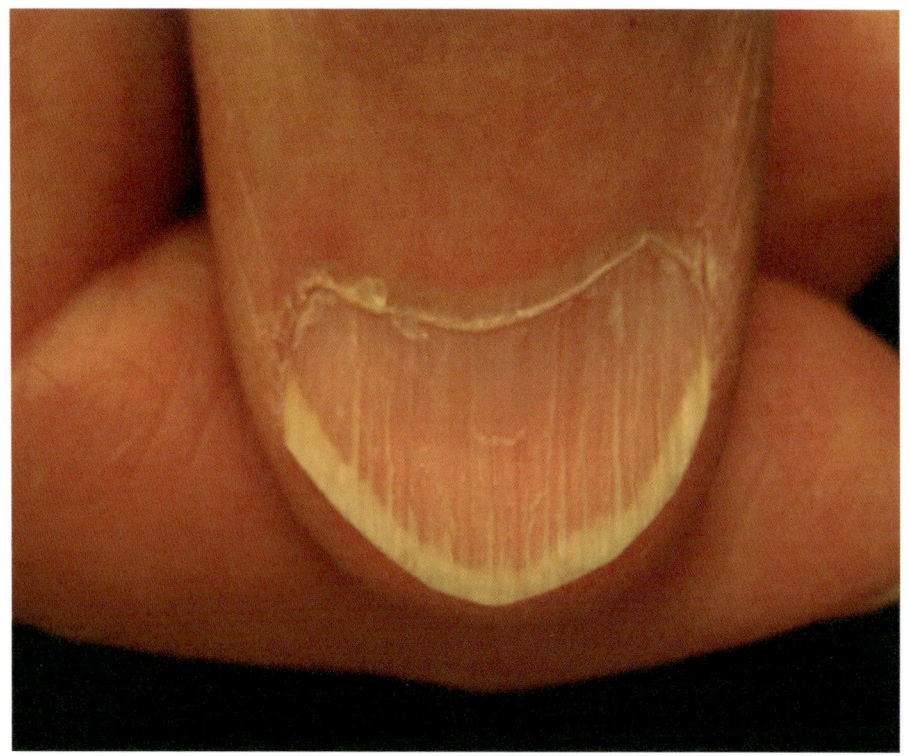

Absent Lunula

ABSENT LUNULA

An absent lunula implies chronic anemia, malnutrition or depression. The thumb is the best place to confirm the finding because if the lunula is present on the thumb an absent lunula on another digit is nonspecific. In fact it is common to see an absent lunula on the little finger with visible lunula on other fingers.

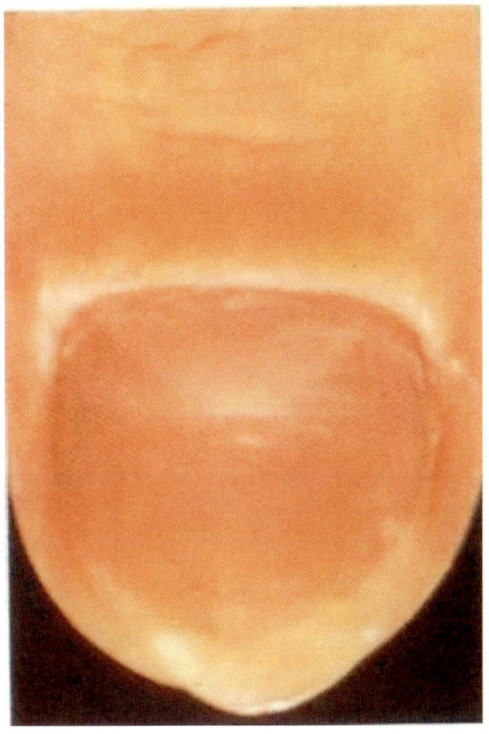

Triangular Lunula

TRIANGULAR LUNULA

Repetitive trauma to the cuticle causes the lunula to lose its gentle curvature becoming more triangular or pyramidal. The repetitive trauma is often related to excessive manicure, habit, or occupational injury. Sometimes fine transverse lines will be seen on the surface as well.

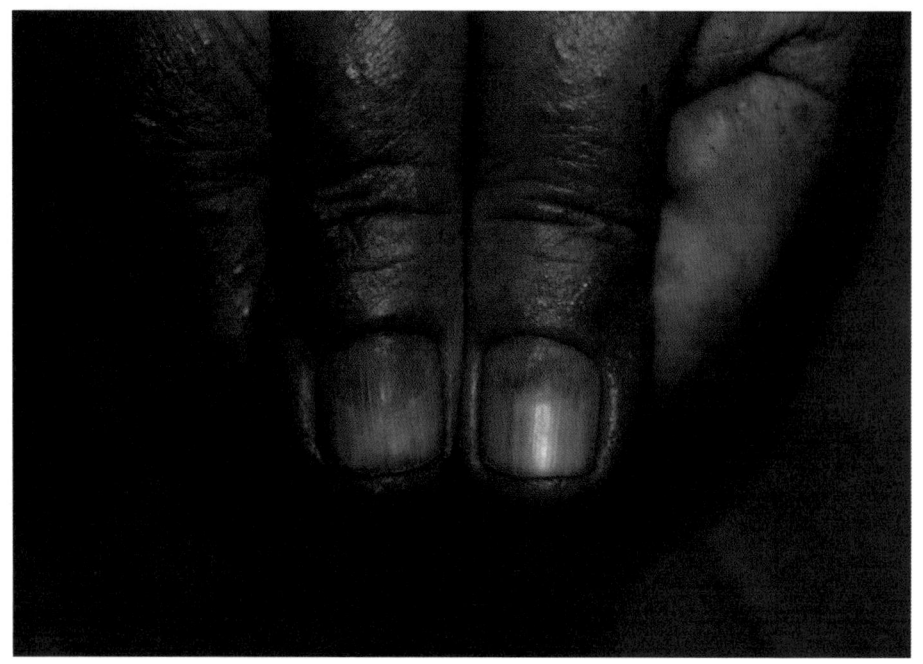

Lunular blush (Red lunula)

LUNULAR BLUSH

A red lunula or lunular blush is sometimes evident when the normal contrast is reduced between the lunula (normally white) and the nail plate (normally pink). It blanches with pressure suggesting that it is caused by vascular dilation of the digital arterioles. A lunular blush is a clue to cardiovascular disease (over 50% of the time) but can also be seen in hematological malignancy and collagen vascular disease.

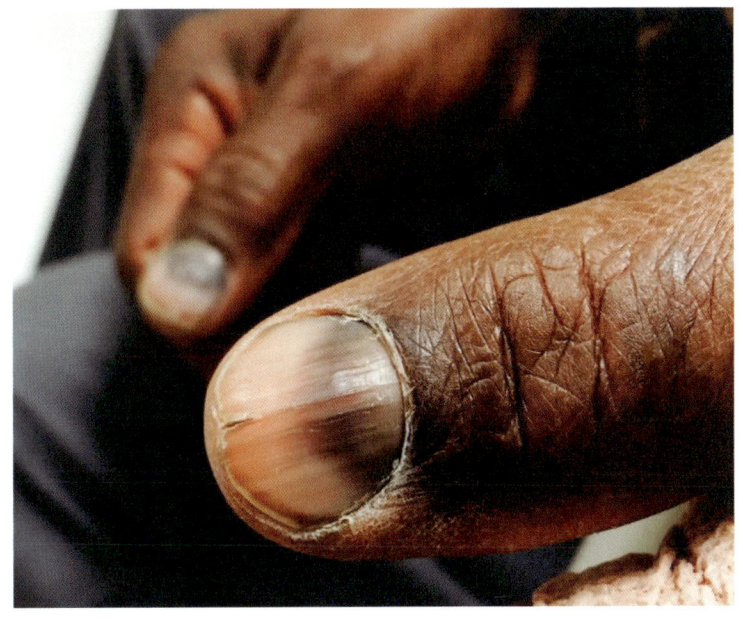

Brown lunula

BROWN LUNULA

Brown pigmentation involving the lunula raises the possibility the person is taking hydroxyurea, which could reflect hematogenous malignancy, essential thrombocytosis, polycythemia rubra vera, sickle cell disease or HIV.

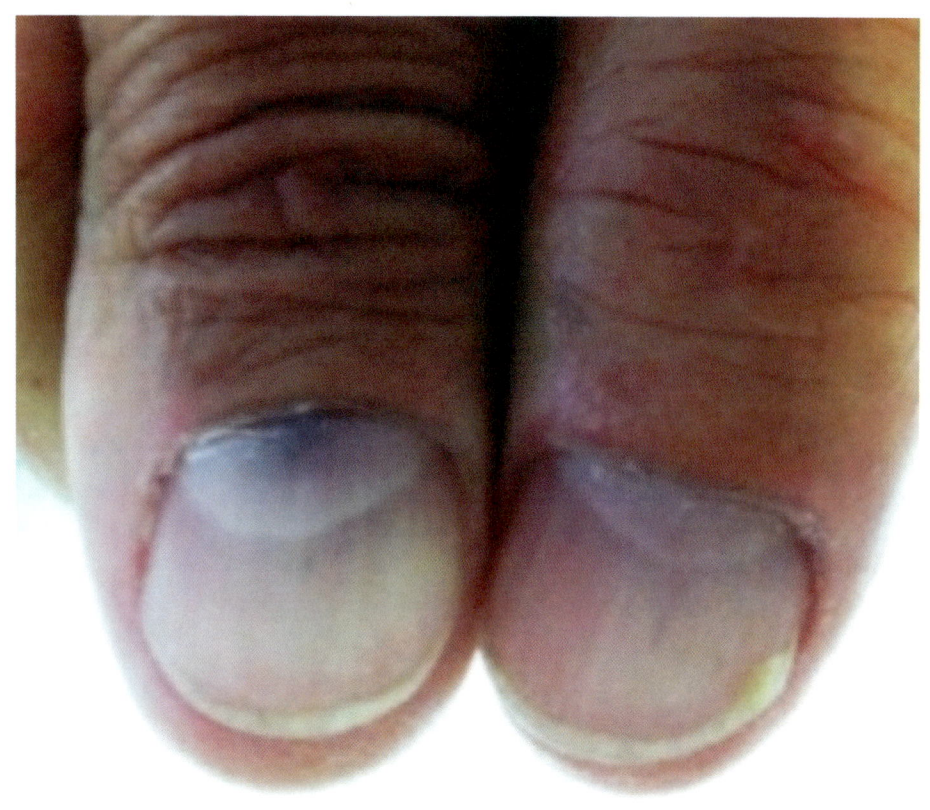

Single black lunula

A discoloration of one lunula suggests a local process such as trauma or malignancy. The normal nail surface and no paronychial bruising makes recent trauma less likely and the lack of pigmentation extending into the matrix reduces the chance of melanoma. In this case the pigmentation was due to a childhood accident with a lead pencil.

BIFID LUNULA (no image)

A very rare lunular manifestation is the bifid lunula. It resembles two camel humps and is associated with polydactyly.

Chapter 3

Abnormalities Of Nail Shape

After noting the lunula, the next basic observation involves the shape of the nails. The goal is to determine if the shape is normal or if an abnormality is present. The first example of an abnormally shaped nail is clubbing.

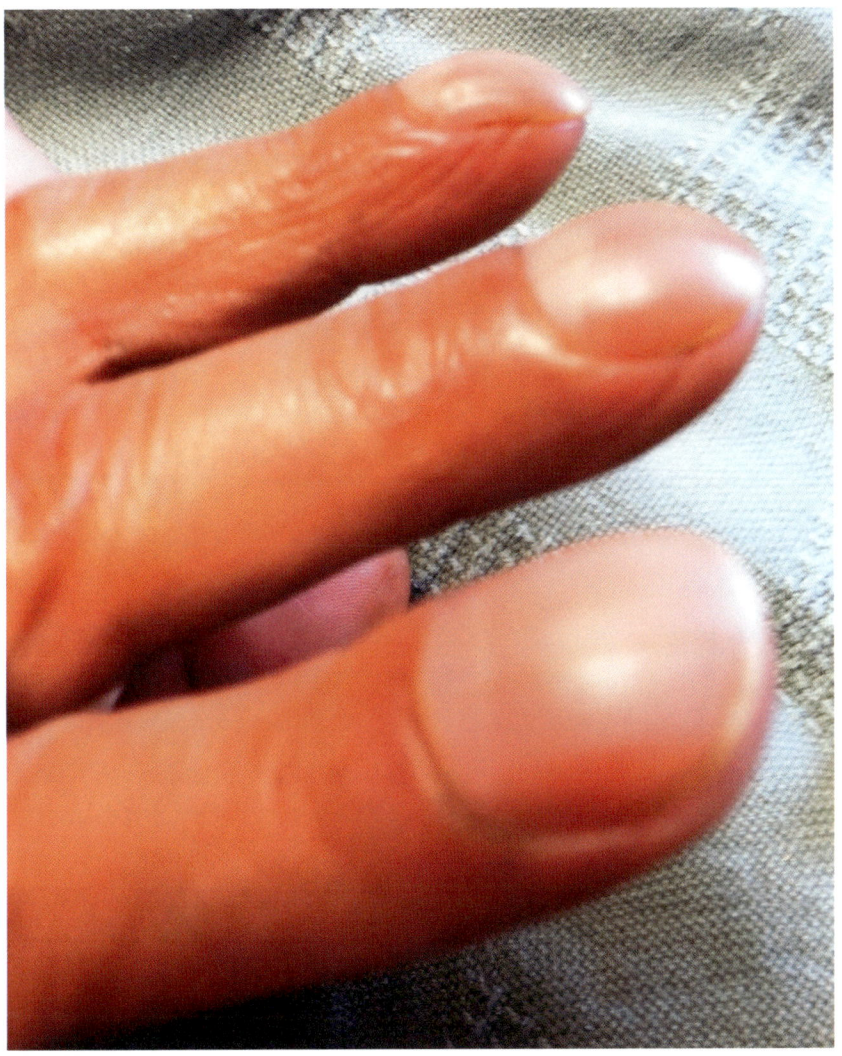

Clubbing

Notice if the fingers are clubbed. The key feature of clubbing is that the distal caliber of the finger is larger than the proximal caliber. In advanced clubbing they will be drumstick-like resembling a caveman's club. (See Image). Nail curvature without the increase in caliber is not clubbing. There are 4 phases of clubbing and the nuances are not important, the key observation is whether the nails are clubbed or not.

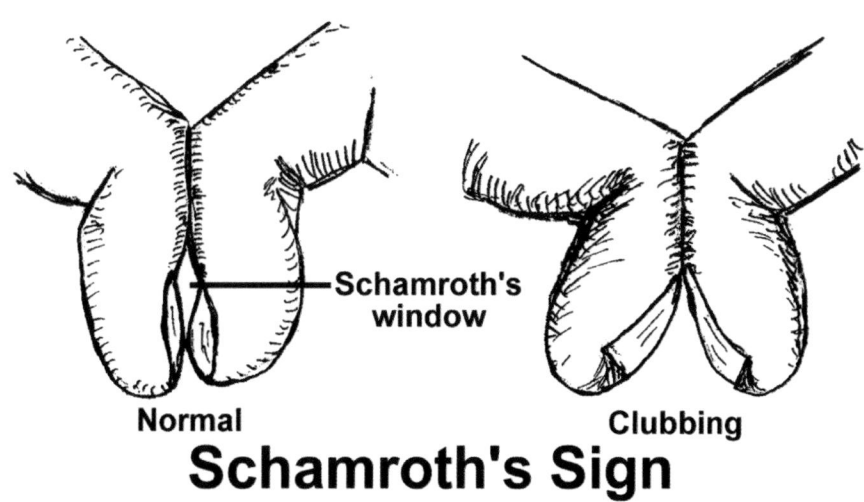

Schamroth's Sign

One of the earliest signs of clubbing is that the nail loses its angle of insertion. To look for loss of this angle check Schamroth's sign: have the patient place both forefinger nails together and look between them. If you can see a small diamond space between them then the nails are not clubbed. Also notice that as the clubbing advances the fingertips point away from each other rather than straight down.

The mechanism of clubbing is not entirely clear (at least to me) although it may involve changes in autonomic control of the digital arterioles that help to modulate body heat. Changes in vasomotor compounds such as kinins and prostaglandins also increase blood flow through the fingertip. The mechanism for clubbing probably varies for differing conditions.

Table Possible Causes of Acquired Clubbing

ORGAN SYSTEM	POSSIBLE CAUSE OF THE CLUBBING
Lung disease	Lung carcinoma
	Alveolar cell carcinoma
	Lung abscess (the condition first associated with clubbing by Hippocrates)
	Interstitial pulmonary fibrosis
	Sarcoidosis
	Beryllium poisoning
Heart disease	Subacute bacterial endocarditis
	Infected arterial grafts
	Aortic aneurysm
Gastrointestinal conditions	Inflammatory bowel disease
	Sprue
	Neoplasms (esophagus, liver, bowel)
Other	Hyperthyroidism

The causes of clubbing are numerous and the Table is not exhaustive. The key point is that pulmonary and cardiovascular causes account for about 80% of clubbing and usually have additional symptoms and signs. The specific diagnosis can sometimes be identified by the additional clues such as splinter hemorrhages in bacterial endocarditis. Gastrointestinal causes are associated with clubbing in 5% of cases. Hyperthyroidism can also produce clubbing (about 1%). Normally I do not consider Grave's disease when I see clubbing. However, in a person with thyrotoxicosis and acquired clubbing I remember that the association is there and I do not have to consider other causes to explain the clubbing unless other clues point toward another diagnosis.

When I appreciate acquired clubbing I tend to think of occult pulmonary or GI malignancy unless other features of illness point to another possibility. It is important to remember that chronic obstructive lung disease (COPD) doe not cause clubbing. When you notice clubbing in a person with COPD look for the underlying cancer.

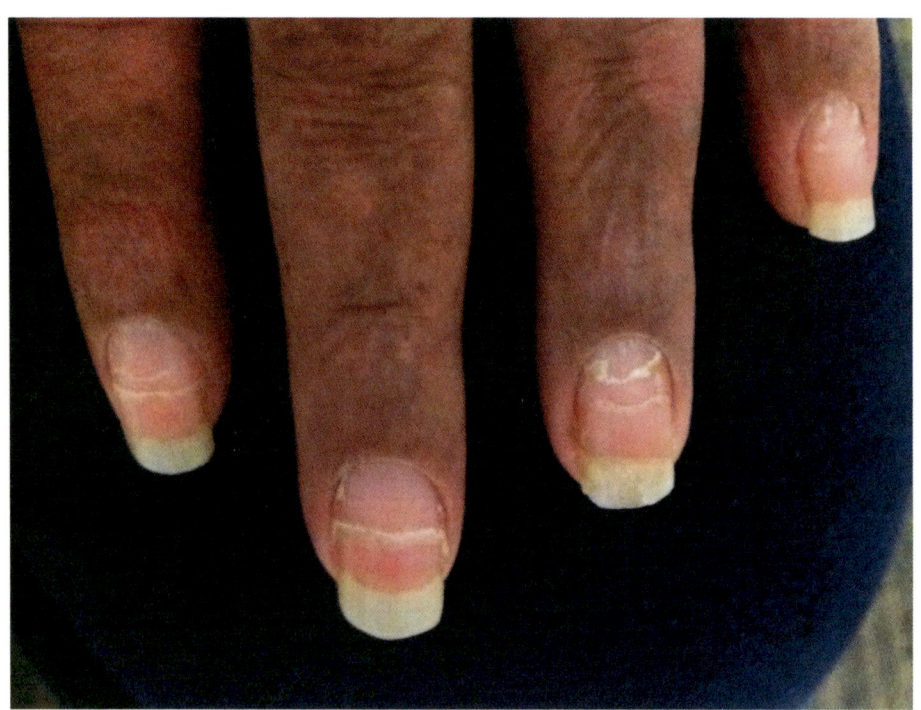

Beau's lines

TRANSVERSE LINES (BEAU'S LINES)

In 1846, a French physician, Joseph Honoré Simon Beau (1806–1865) described transverse lines in the substance of the nail as signs of previous acute illness. By noting its location on the nail the approximate date of the illness can be determined. In the image above the Beau's line is approximately one half of the way up the nail suggests significant acute illnesses 3 months ago (since it takes six months for the nail to fully grow out. Moreover the depth of the line provides a clue to the severity of the illness. The mechanism appears to be an illness severe enough to stop or slow down nail production.

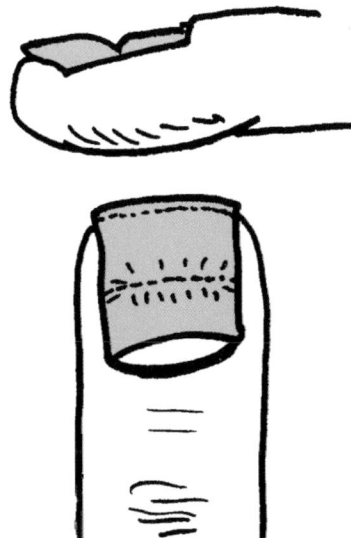

Beau's Growth Arrest Line

The lines look as if a little furrow had been plowed across the nail.

Illnesses producing Beau's lines include severe infection,

myocardial infarction, hypotension, shock, or surgery. Intermittent doses of immunosuppressive therapy or chemotherapy can also produce Beau's growth arrest lines. Severe zinc deficiency has also been proposed as a cause of Beau's lines.

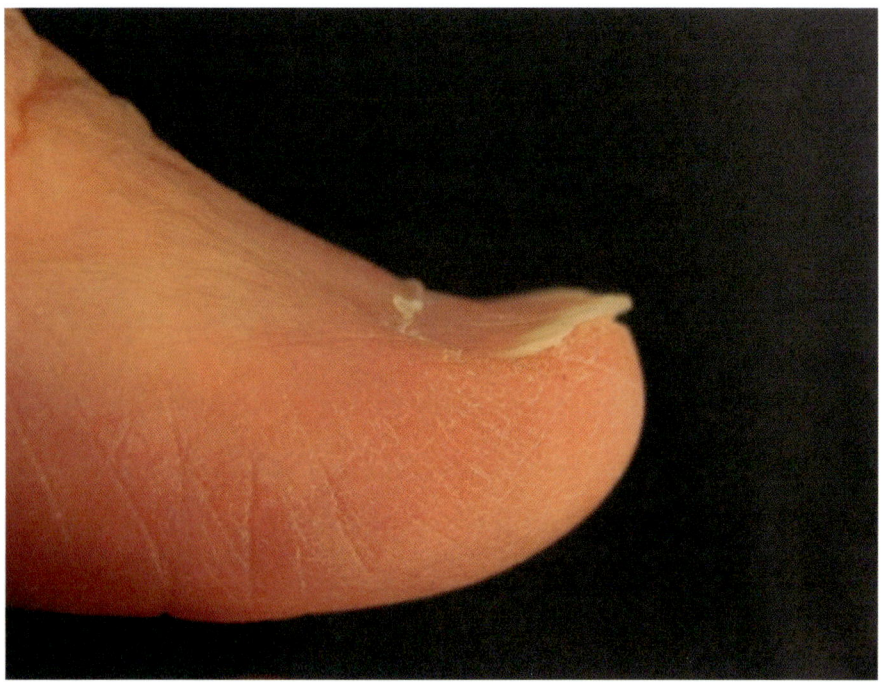

Spoon nails

KOILONYCHIA (SPOON NAILS)

Koilonychia gets its name from "koilos" which is the Greek word for spoon. The nail shape changes from mildly convex to frankly concave (See image). When you see a spoon nail think "nutrient deficiency." Spoon nails suggest iron deficiency, protein deficiency, or deficiency in sulfur-containing amino acids (cysteine or methionine). The thickness of the nail plate can help you to infer the underlying disorder.

Soft, thin spoon nails are seen in iron deficiency and deficiency of amino acids. Since small amounts of insulin and growth hormone are necessary for amino acid transport, uncontrolled diabetes (hemoglobin A1C over 10) can produce koilonychias with thick nails. Rarely, spoon nails can be seen in Raynaud's phenomenon.

To determine if a nail is spooned perform the water drop test. Place a drop of water on the nail. If the drop does not slide off then the nail is flattened from early spooning. With practice you should be able to look at the nail and perform a "mental" water drop test.

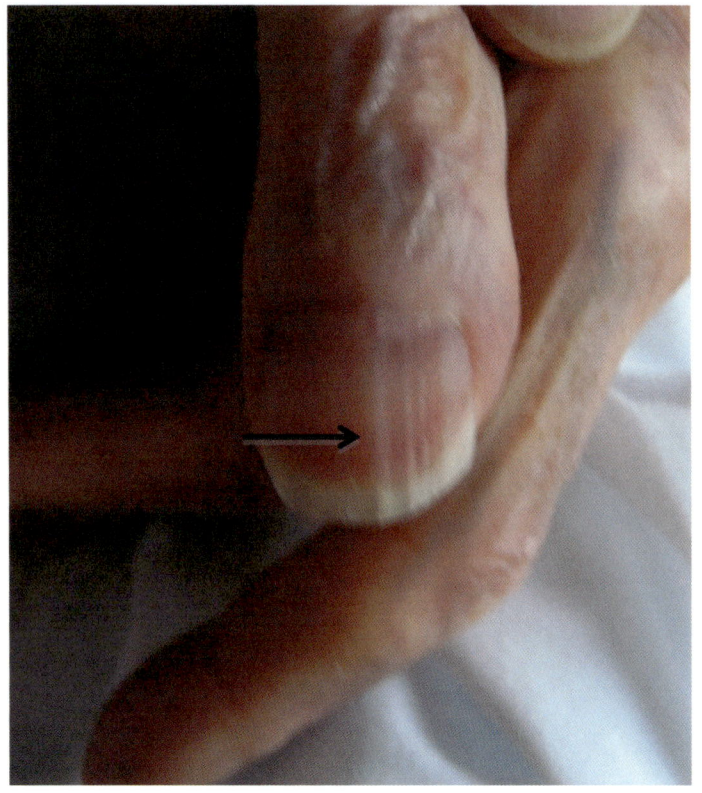

Central ridge

CENTRAL RIDGE

A central thin ridge can be seen in iron, folic acid, or protein deficiency. When you see a central ridge think "nutrient deficiency." There are two varieties of central nail ridging but the significance is the same. The first variant has a bar running down the nail and looks like the keel of a boat (See image).

The second variant looks like two shallow spoons with a ridge in between. The mechanism producing the central ridge may relate to the blood supply to the matrix that forms an arteriolar net-work from the digital arteries. Nutrients are delivered from the sides and diffuse into the center of the matrix. With normal blood flow the central portion of the nail gets nutrition from each side (relatively more than the neighboring cells on the edges). As a result, nutrient deficiency affects the cells on the edges more than the centrally located cells.

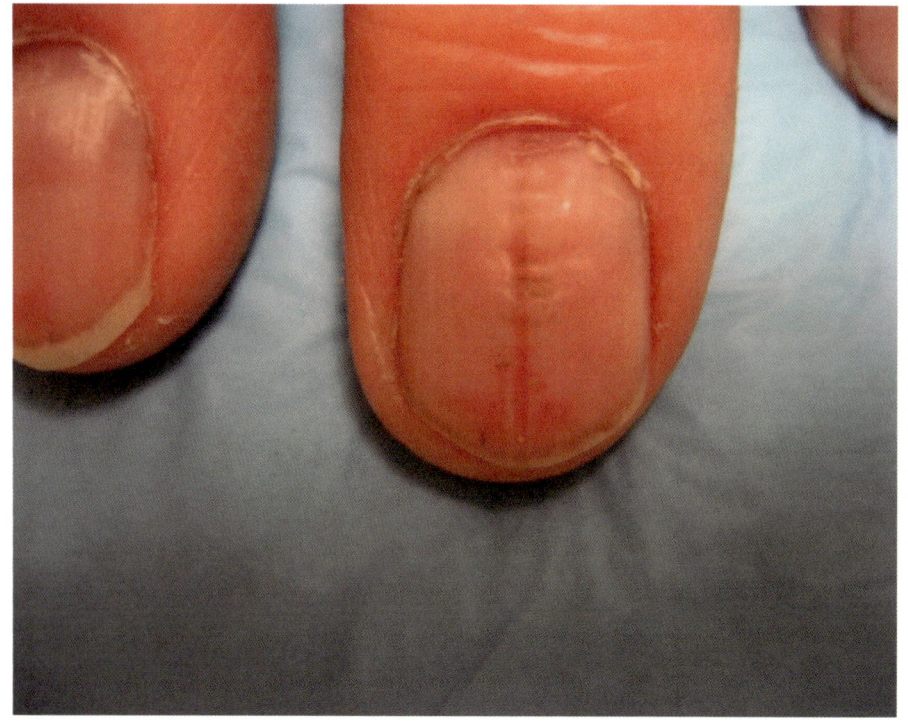

Central canal

CENTRAL CANAL (MEDIAN NAIL DYSTROPHY)

A central nail canal is sometimes called "Median Nail Dystrophy." It appears as a longitudinal pink line (sometimes called "Heller's line") or an actual longitudinal defect in the nail.

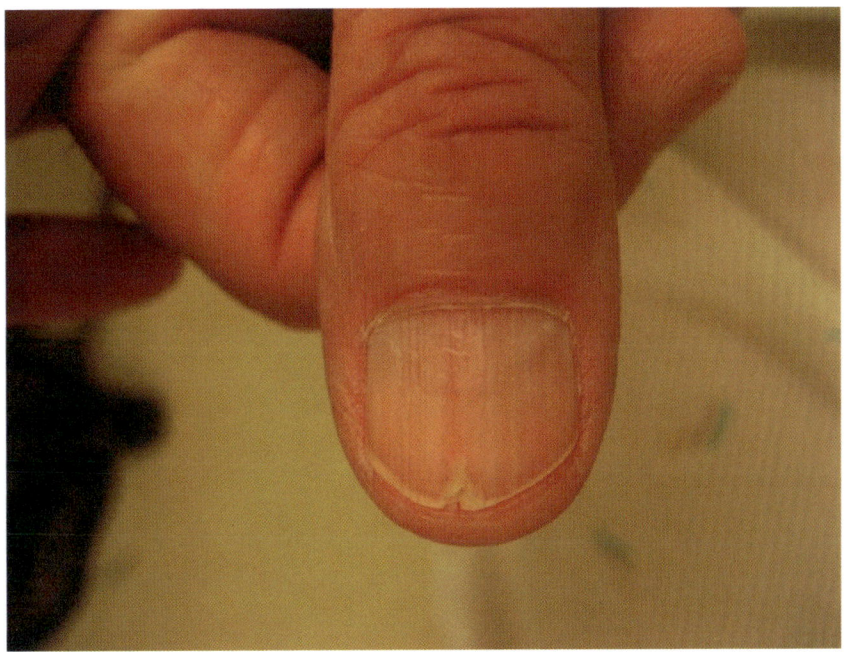

Central canal with indentation

Occasionally there will be an indention at the tip of the nail. The mechanism is severe peripheral arterial disease, severe malnutrition, or repetitive trauma to the cuticle. Since the central cells in the nail matrix are in a nutritional watershed area they are vulnerable to chronic vascular insufficiency or profound malnutrition.

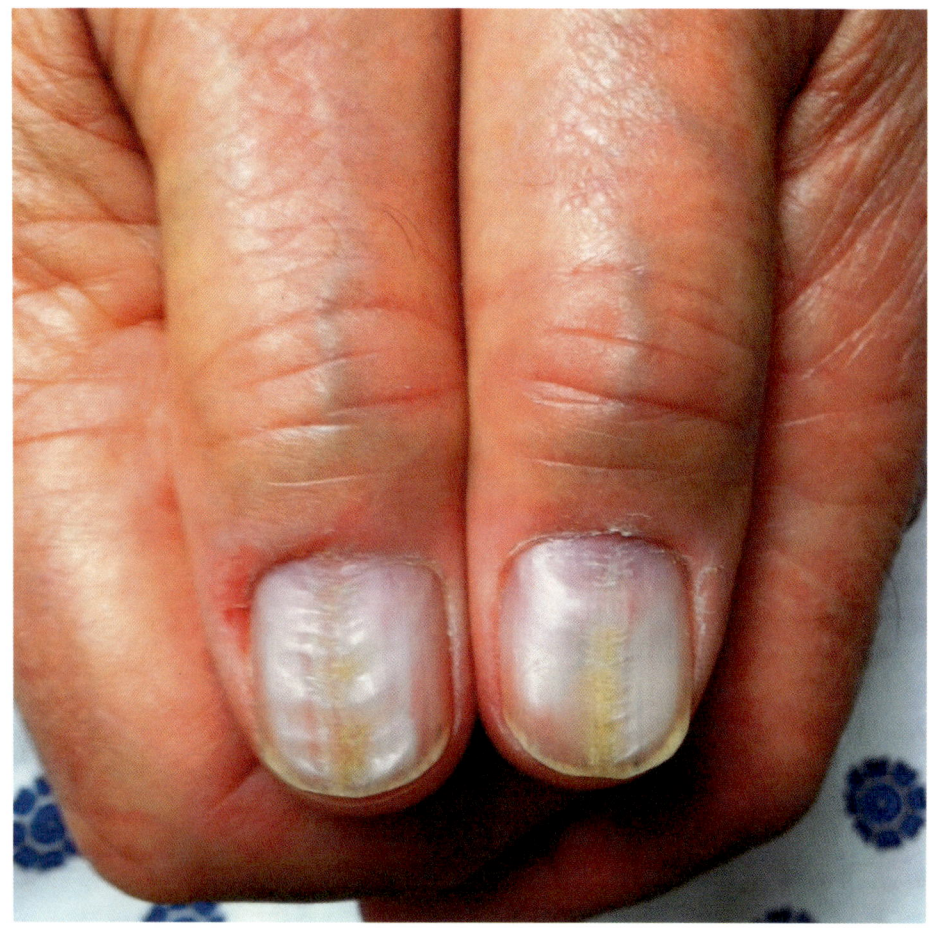

Heller's deformity

Repetitive cuticular trauma may scar the underlying vasculature producing relative ischemia. Fine transverse lines from the trauma called "Heller's deformity" can be seen occasionally.

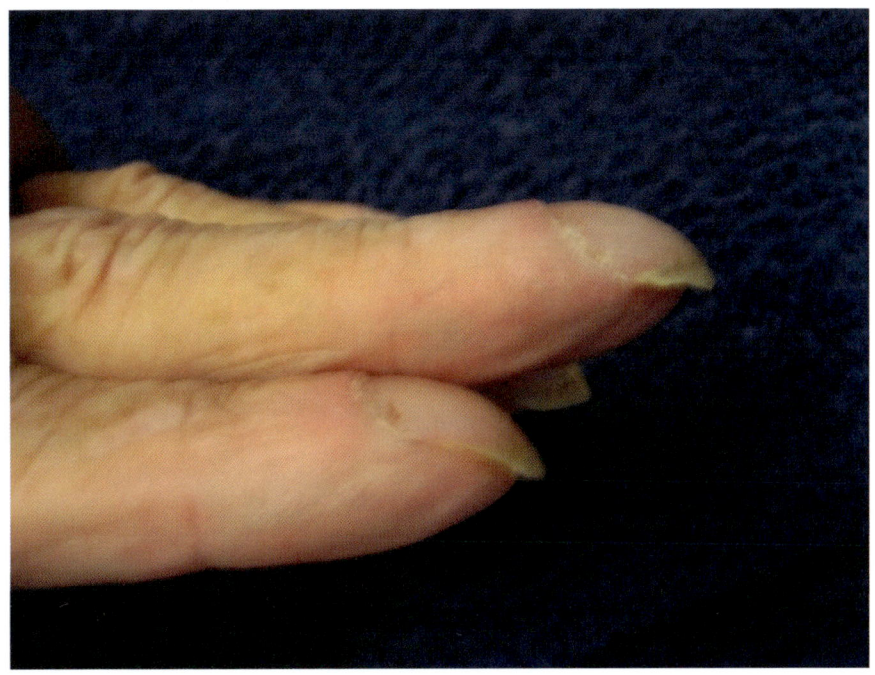

Beaked nails

BEAKED NAILS

Excessively curved nails are sometimes called "beaked nails" because they resemble a bird's beak. Notice that the distal caliber of the finger is not larger than the proximal caliber so the nails are not really clubbed.

The mechanism of curved nails is resorption of the distal digit. Conditions that can resorb the distal digits are primary hyperparathyroidism, renal failure with secondary hyperparathyroidism, malignancy with hyperparathyroidism (usually squamous cell cancers producing PTHrP), psoriasis, and systemic sclerosis.

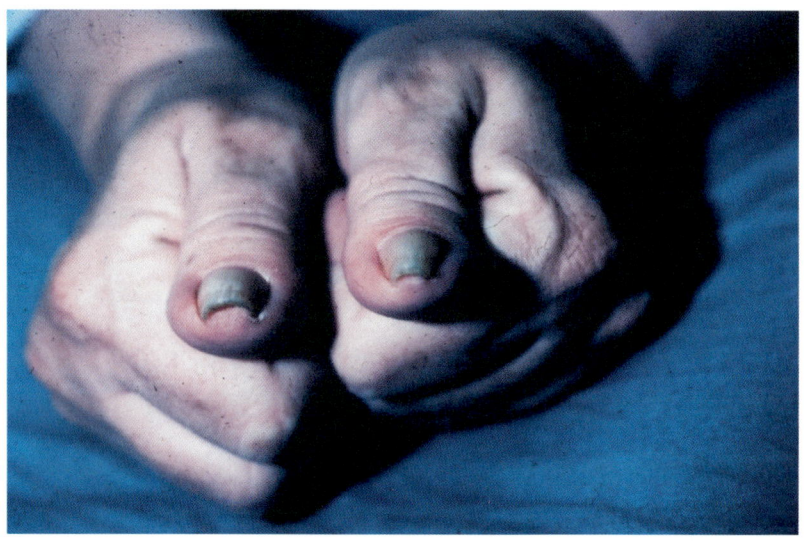

Pincer nails

PINCER NAILS

Ingrown nails are rounded along the sides creating a rolled appearance. They can result from nails being cut too short or clipping the edge too far down the side of the nail. Over time these nails can predispose to swelling and infection (paronychia).

Chapter 4

Abnormalities Of The Nail Surface

The surface of the fingernail can reveal important clues to metabolic bone disease, nail growth rate, habits, occupational exposures, as well as signs of systemic diseases such as endocrine disorders, and systemic vasculitis.

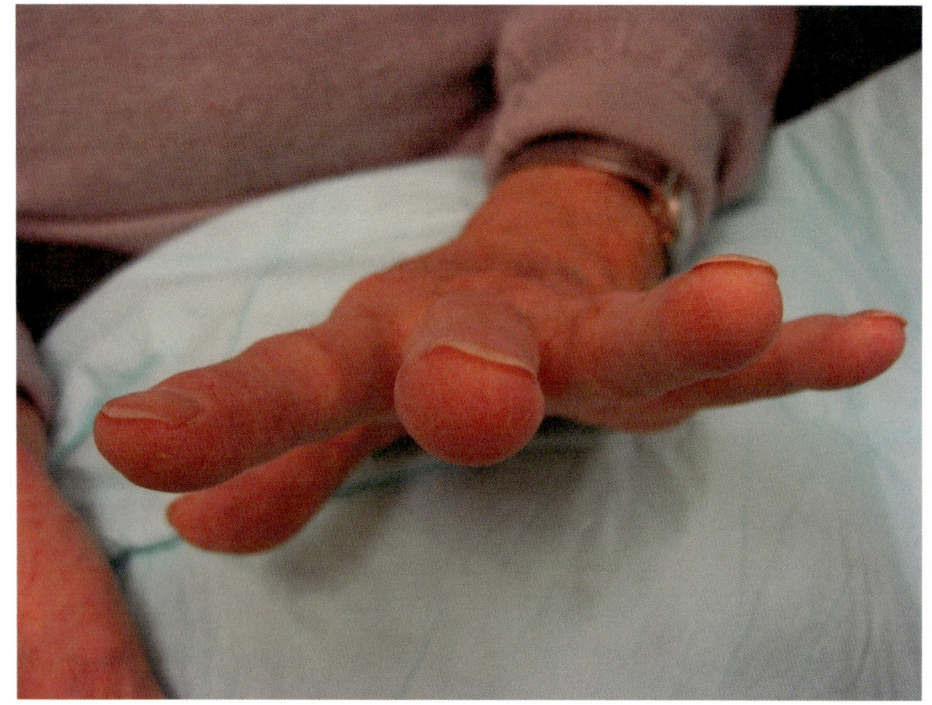

Thin nails

THIN BRITTLE NAILS

Notice the very ends of the nails, head on, to determine how thick they appear. These nails look normal from the top down but are tissue paper thin when viewed on end. The implication is metabolic bone disease. There is a direct linear correlation between the thickness of the fingernails and the amount of calcium in the skeleton. The thinner the nails the less bone. Some experts have used a micrometer to measure nail thickness.

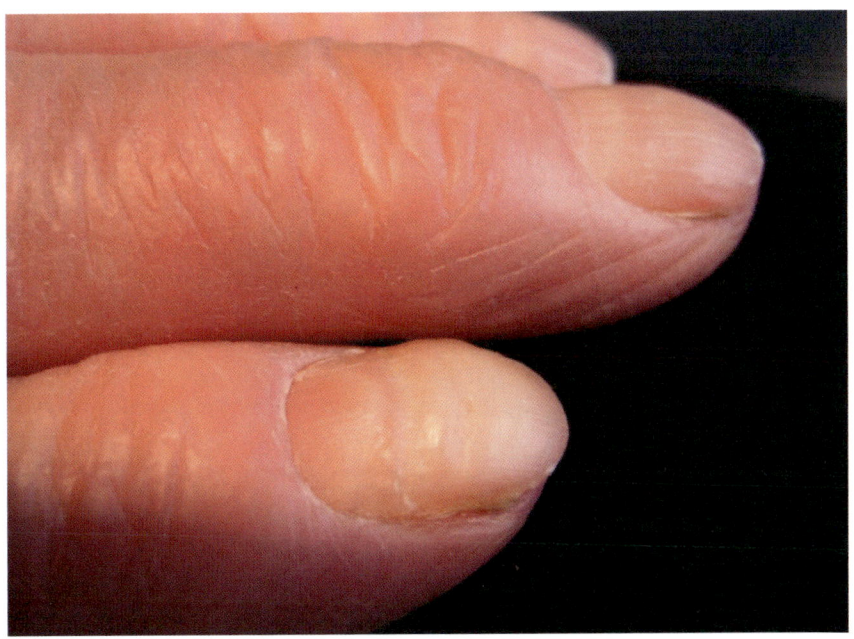

Thick nails

NAIL THICKENING

The mechanism of nail thickening is slowing of the growth rate. Conditions that can slow the growth rate are fungal disease (onychomycosis), chronic eczema, peripheral vascular disease, psoriasis, and yellow nail syndrome. The nails in the photo were in a patient with peripheral vascular disease. (Did you notice the red lunula implying heart disease and the two Beau's lines showing acute illness?)

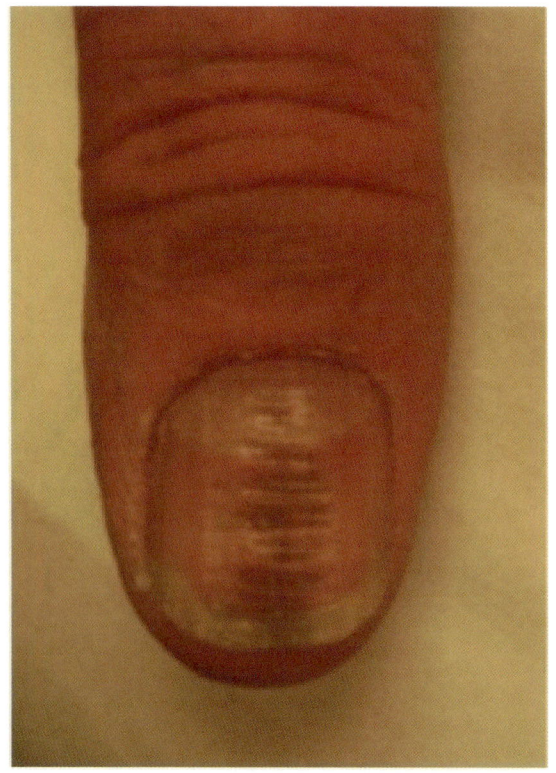

Transverse lines

TRANSVERSE LINES

Irregular transverse lines represent repetitive trauma to the cuticle most often caused by occupational injury or habit. They tend to be on one or two nails. Occasionally there will be dark coloration from dirt or other exposure. In the case above the lines cover the entire nail length indicating constant trauma.

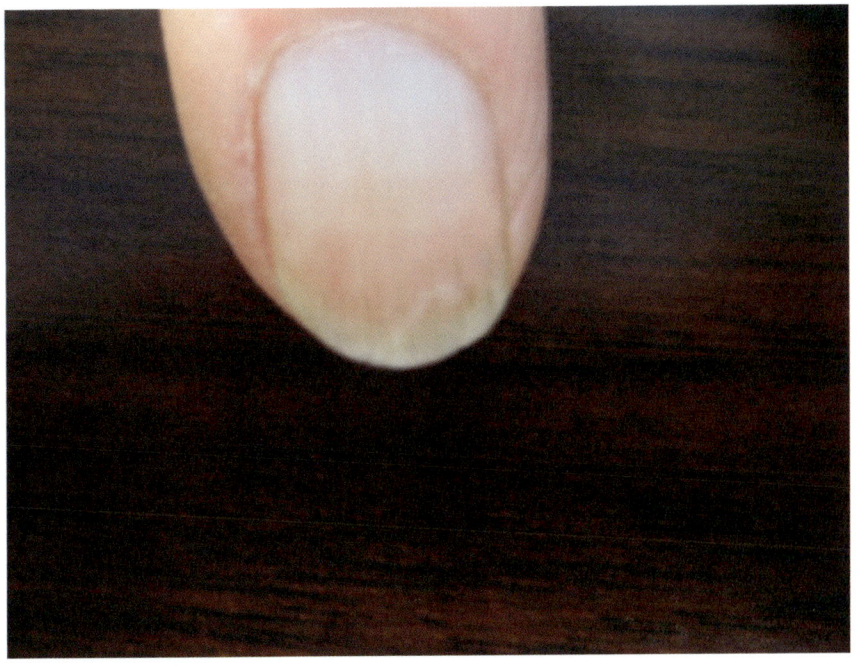

Brittle nail tip

BRITTLE NAIL TIPS

These nails suggest thyroid disorder (usually hyperthyroidism) or malnutrition. Note the pallor and loss of lunula in the photo.

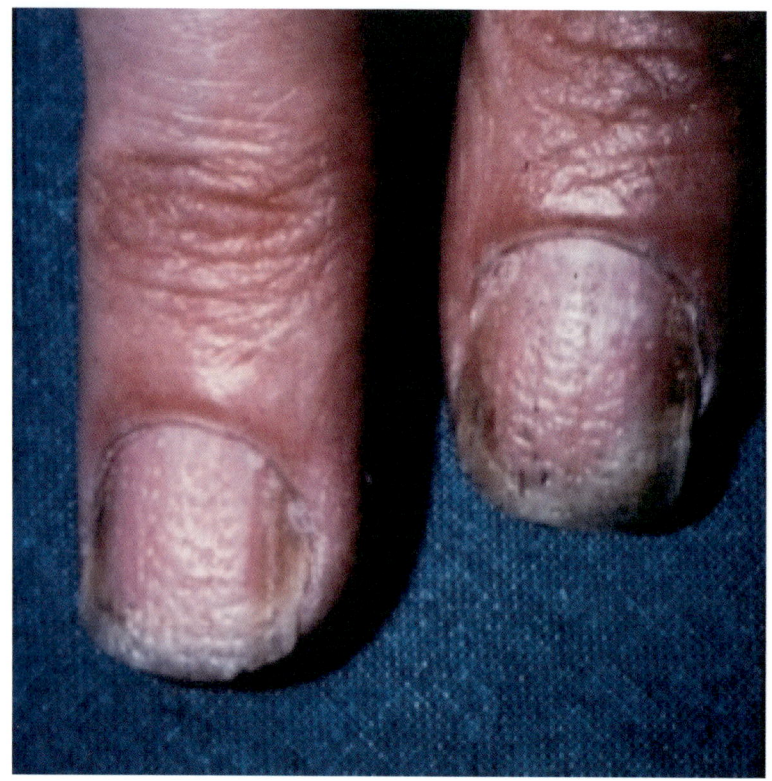

Nail pitting (alopecia areata)

NAIL PITTING

Nail pitting is the presence of numerous fine pits it the nail surface resembling pinpricks. The mechanism is nail matrix inflammation (so the matrix below the cuticle often looks puffy and red). These nails are associated with dermatological conditions: psoriasis, alopecia areata, eczema, and lichen planus.

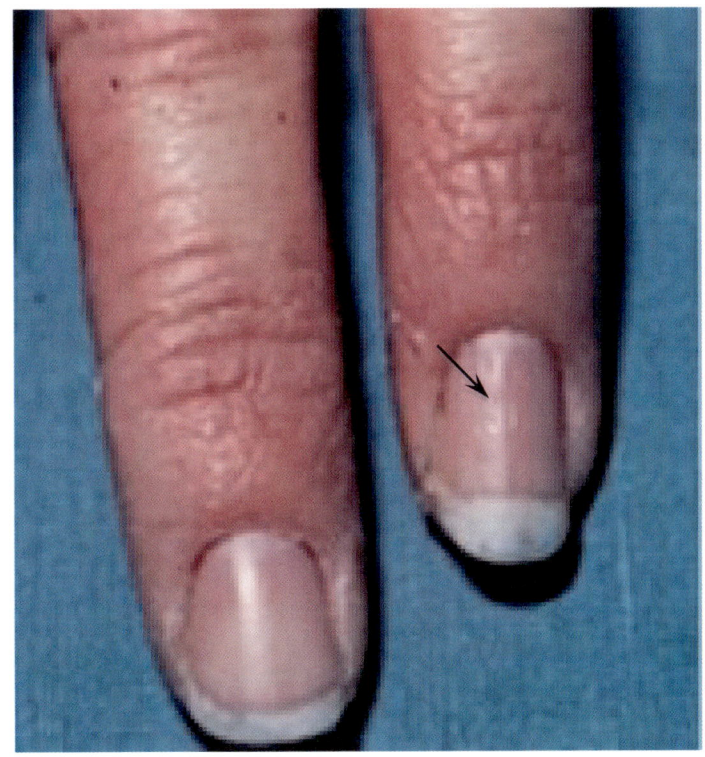

Psoriatic pitting (random pits)

Normally the associated dermatological condition is obvious and the source of the pitting is clear. However in early illness the nail findings may be the most visible clue. The geometry of the pitting can have diagnostic utility: in psoriasis the pitting appears scattered and random while it is much denser in alopecia areata (See Images).

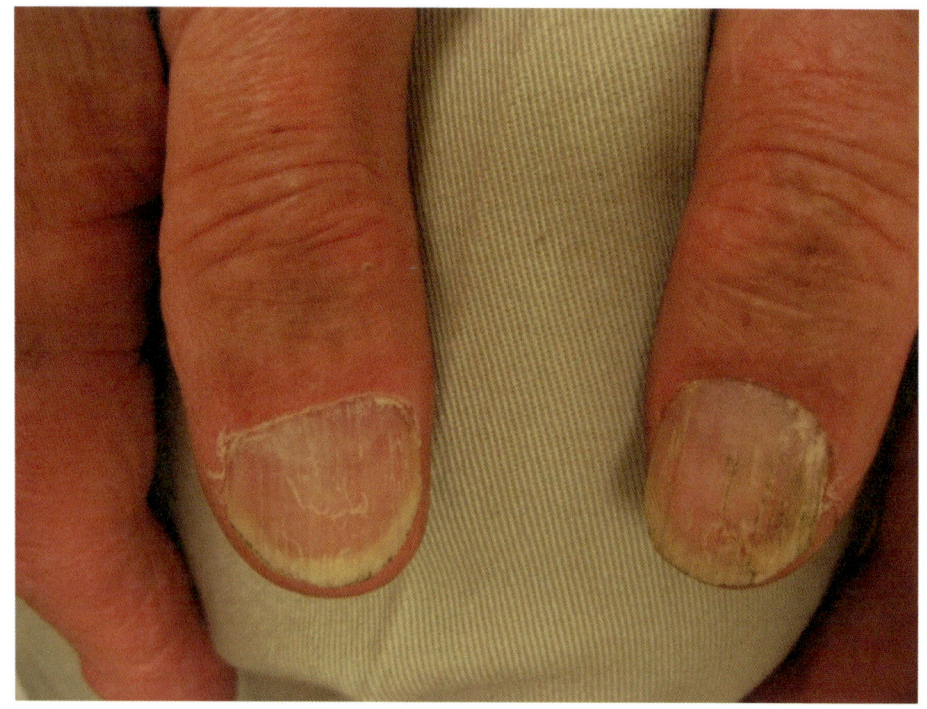

Friable brittle nails

FRIABLE BRITTLE NAILS

These nails look dull and rough. They can be caused by chemical exposures (particularly solvents), autoimmune disease, psoriasis (which can do just about anything to a nail), and lichen planus. Mild fungal disease and superficial trauma are also on the differential diagnosis of rough, brittle nails. If the nails are waxy and yellow or brown consider systemic amyloidosis.

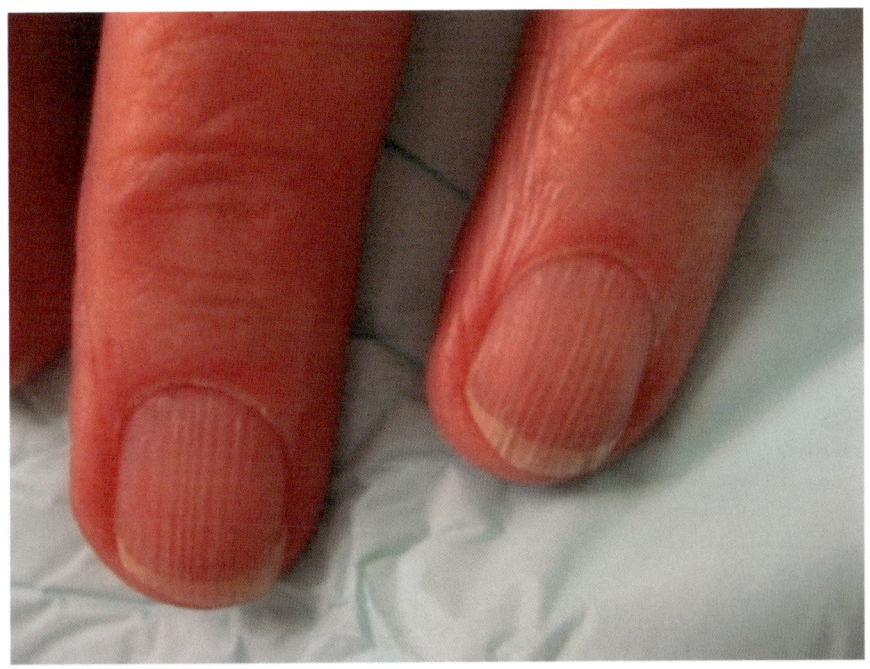

Nail beading

NAIL BEADING

Nail beading refers to longitudinal ridges extending down all the nails. On closer inspection the ridges resemble drips of candle wax. The mechanism may relate to the integrity of the vascular supply and the nature of the capillary network. Nail beading tends to be associated with endocrine disorders and vascular disease. Notice the absent lunula in the nail photo of this woman with diabetes mellitus.

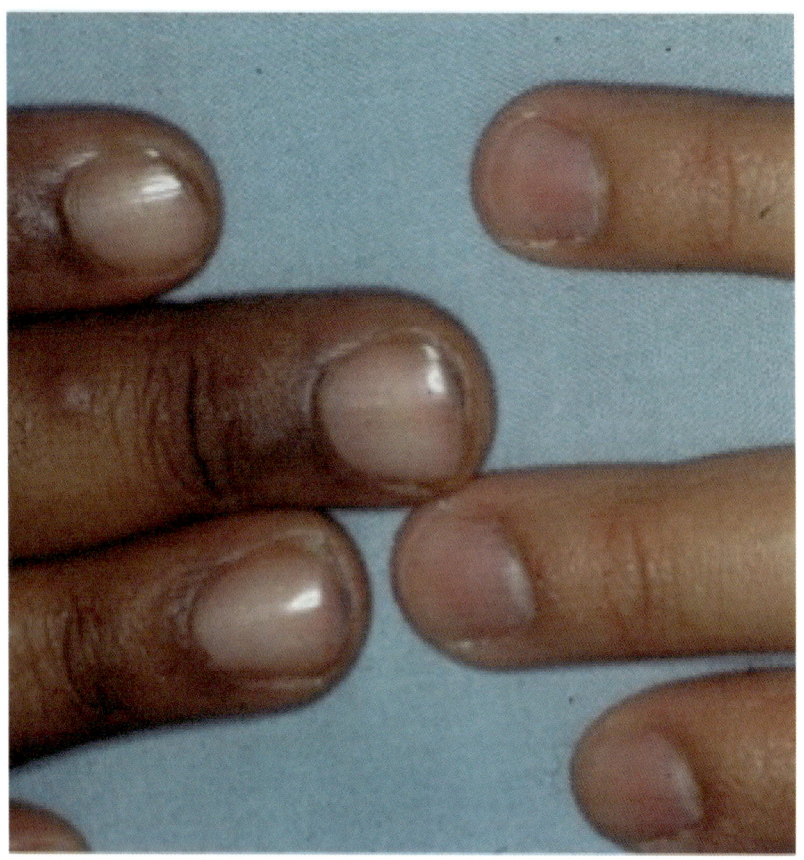

Eburnation

Shiny nails (not resulting from a recent manicure or acrylic nail polish) are called eburnation. They result from significant scratching that burnishes the nails to a luster.

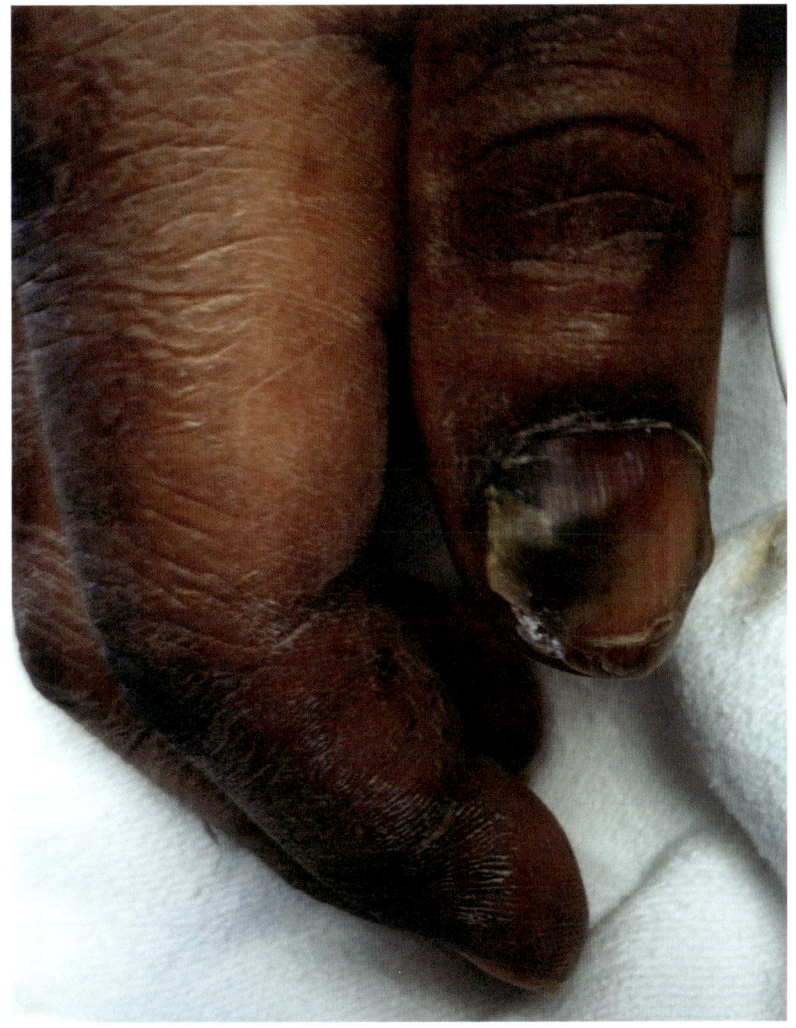

Complete nail destruction

GENERALIZED NAIL DESTRUCTION

This impressive nail looks as if a firecracker was placed under nail and ignited. The nail plate is ragged, disrupted and hemorrhagic.

Sometimes there is paronychial involvement. Like other nail conditions, nail destruction can localized to one or two nails or generalized involving all the nails. Local mechanisms are trauma or infection (paronychias). Generalized nail destruction can be a manifestation of fairly obvious dermatological conditions such as toxic epidermal necrolysis, bullous diseases, or chemotherapy. Another important cause is systemic vasculitis especially polyarteritis nodosa.

Chapter 5

Separation From The Nail Bed

ONYCHOLYSIS

The medical term for separation of the nail from the distal nail plate is onycholysis. The free edge of the nail migrates down toward the cuticle. There are four basic variations: local separation, smooth generalized separation, smooth generalized separation with blistering, and irregular separation.

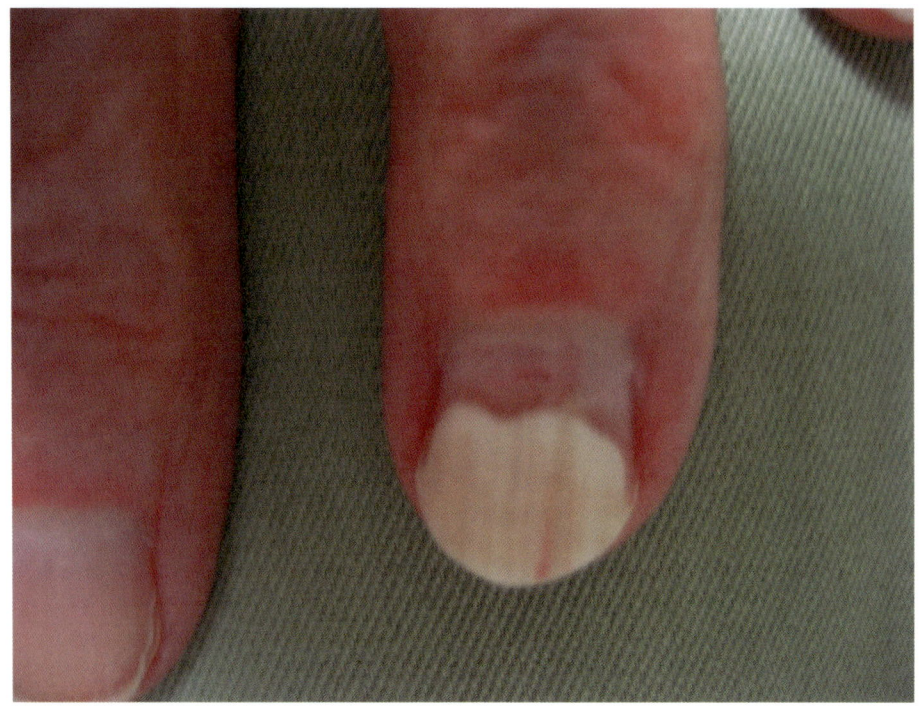

Local Onycholysis (trauma)

In localized onycholysis only a few nails are involved. These nails can be caused by trauma (avulsion), contact dermatitis, toxic exposures (often solvents) fungal disease (onychomycosis) and psoriasis.

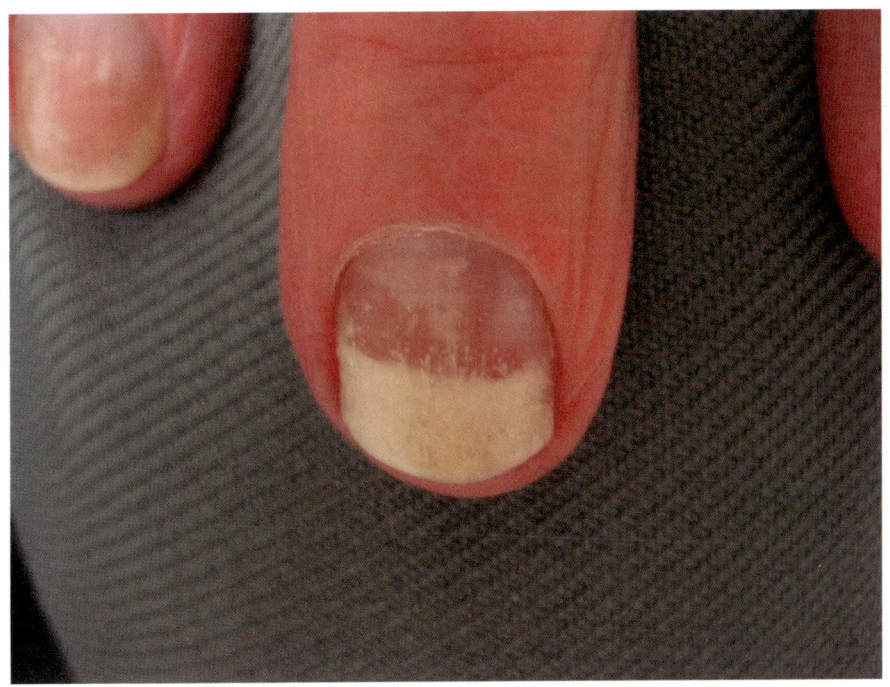

Local Onycholysis (fungal)

In local onycholysis caused by fungi (onychomycosis) the nail can have a chalky white appearance with a fluffy edge to the separation of the nail from the nail plate.

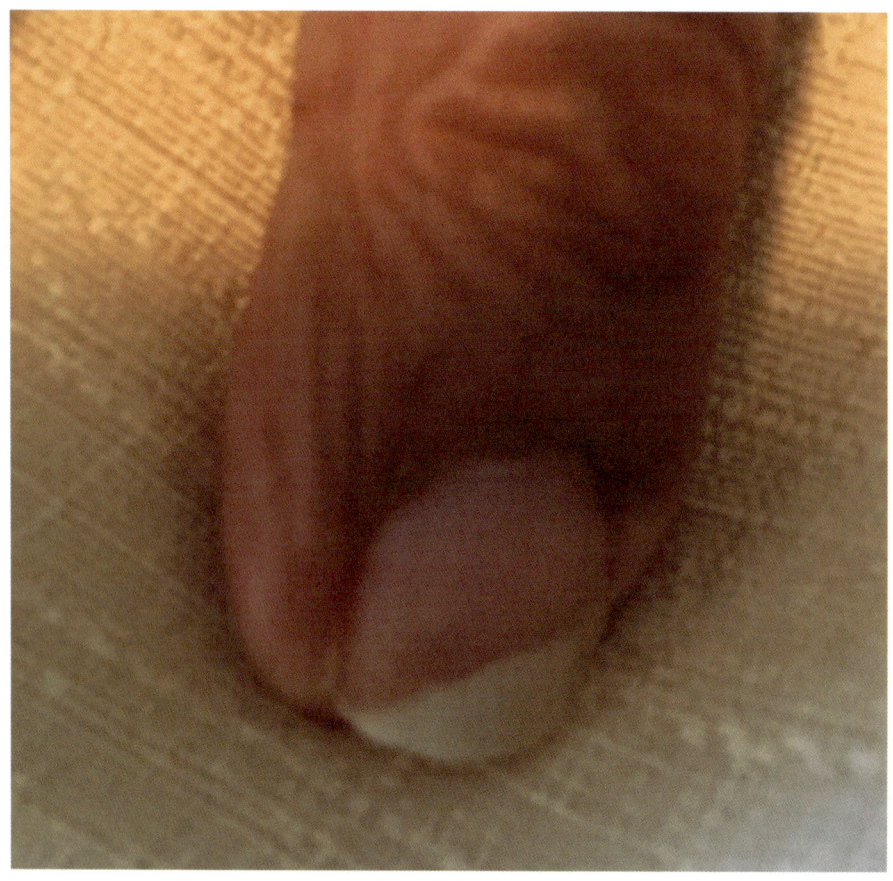

Diagonal Onycholysis

The image shows a diagonal free edge with mild onycholysis from old trauma.

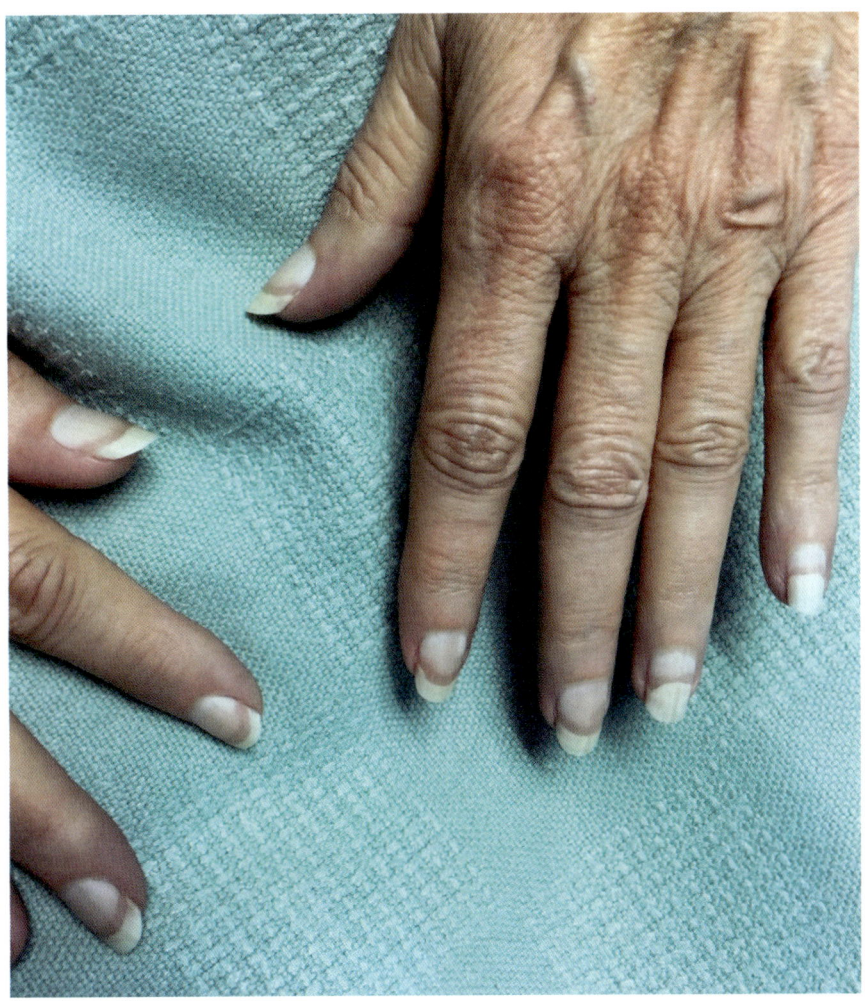

Generalized smooth onycholysis

If all the nails show onycholysis then note the nature of the separation from the nail plate. It will either be smooth or grossly irregular. Most commonly, smooth generalized onycholysis reflects thyrotoxicosis, drug effect (especially tetracyclines), and chemical exposures. Sometimes anemia can produce onycholysis. The example in the figure is subtle but characteristic. The ends of the nails may also be brittle.

If there is also blistering of sun-exposed skin (over the fingers or the dorsum of the wrist) strongly consider porphyria cutanea tarda (PCT). Remember that PCT is one of the cutaneous manifestations of hepatitis C so it is not as rare as it used to be.

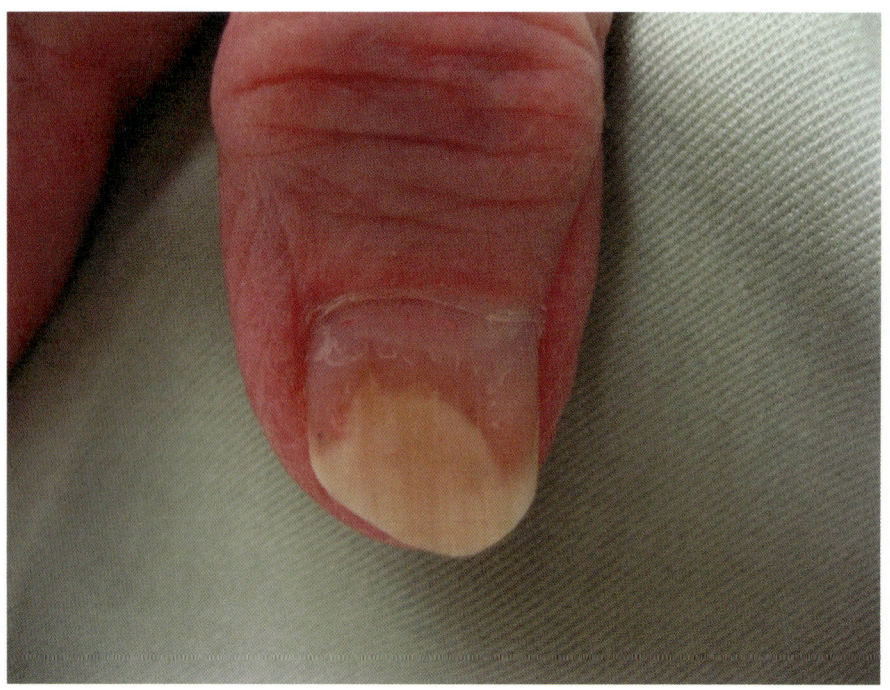

Psoriatic irregular onycholysis

Jagged, irregular separation of the free edge of the nail is characteristic for psoriasis. The nails can vary in involvement and can mimic onychomycosis. Look for other fingernail clues of psoriasis such as pitting, a salmon patch of discoloration in the nail, chronic paronychial inflammation, or inflammation of the matrix.

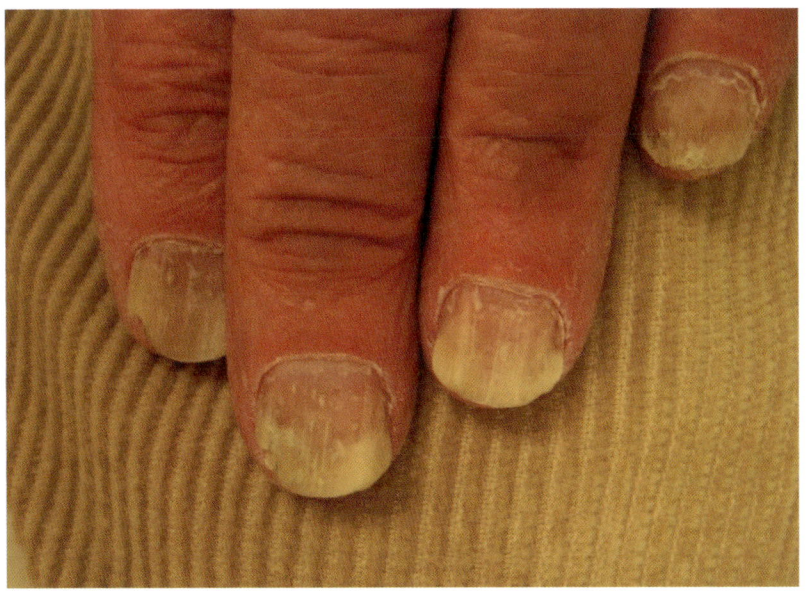

Onychomycosis (Irregular onycholysis)

Onychomycosis is a common nail condition that can also produce irregular onycholysis caused by a fungal infection of the nail. As mentioned above, onychomycosis can produce fluffy powdery, chalk-like discolorations along the nail plate.

CHAPTER 6

Focal Discolorations of the Nail

TRANSVERSE WHITE LINES

Any acute illness can produce transverse milky white lines called Mee's lines if in the setting of arsenic poisoning and Reil's lines in the setting of infection. The mechanism is the failure to lose the nuclei in the cells as the nail is formed. Columns of these nucleated cells produce the milky white discoloration that disappears when the illness abates.

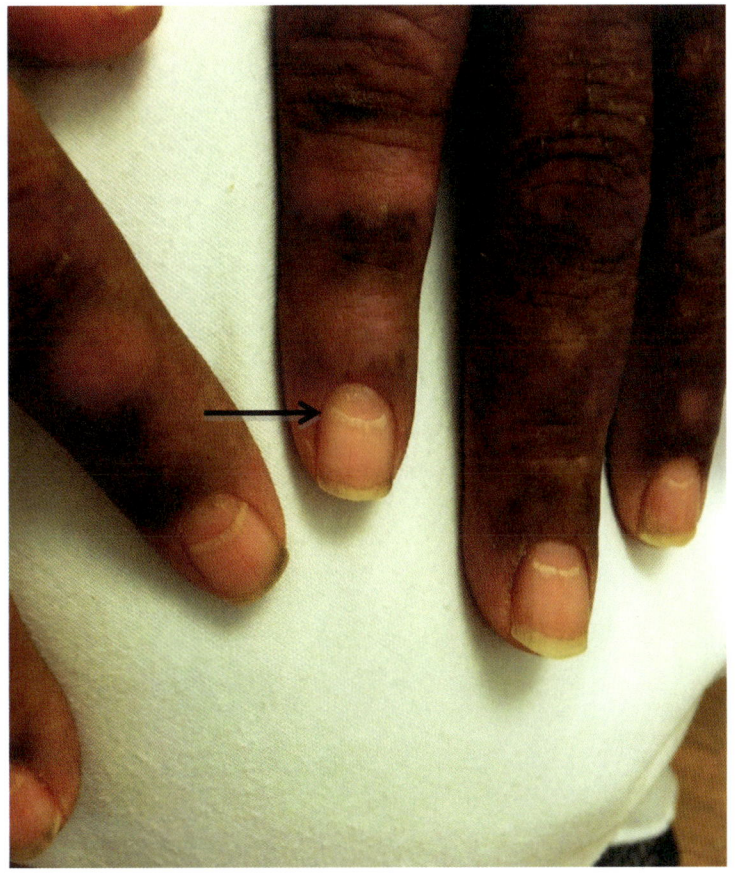

Mees' lines

The timing of the illness can be inferred by the position of the lines on the nails. In the image above the lines are almost one third way up the nail suggesting an illness six weeks to two months ago (since it takes approximately six months for a nail to grow from the cuticle to the free edge). Sometimes a "ladder" of regularly spaced white lines can suggest regular cycles of chemotherapy.

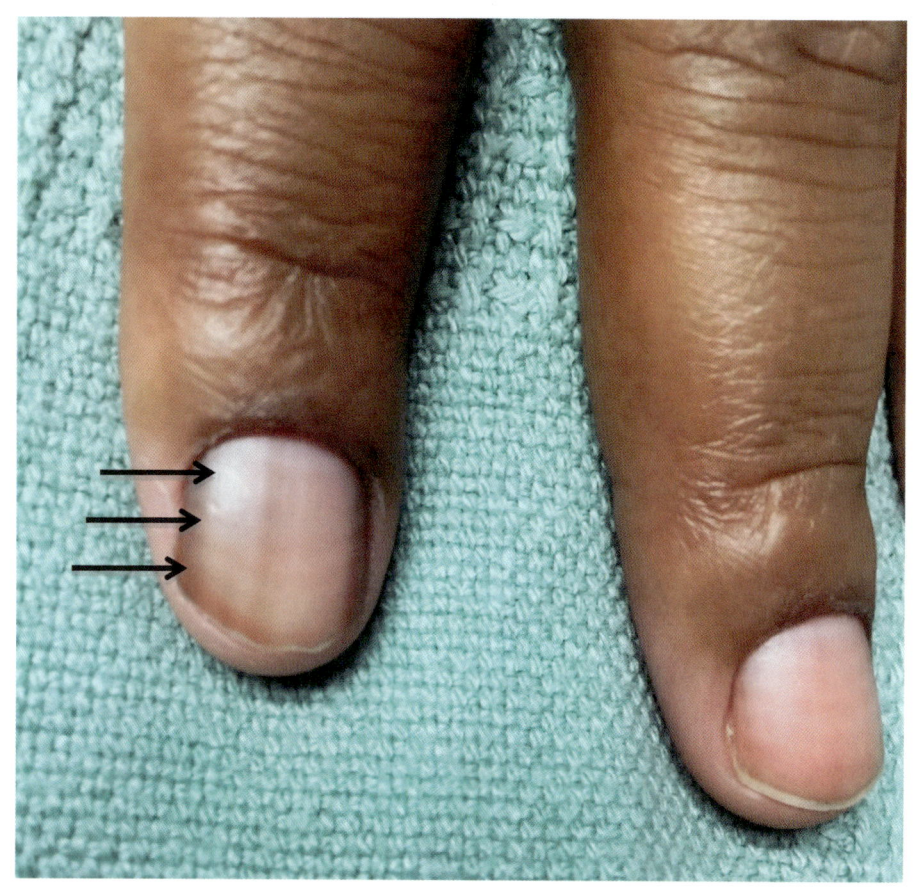

Mees' Ladder

Note the pale transverse lines

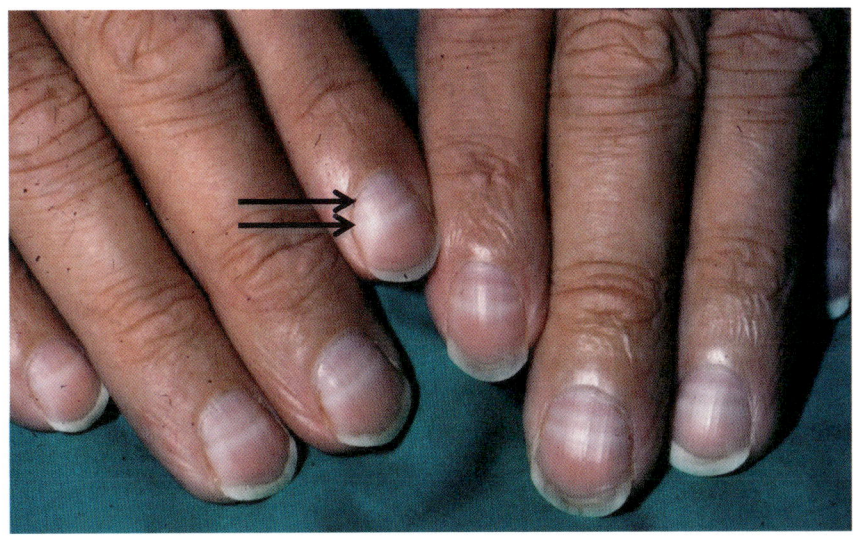

Muehrckes' lines

Muehrckes' lines are irregular parallel white lines caused by very low serum albumin. Edema under the nail produces Muehrcke's lines and they disappear when the albumin rises. Because the lines are not in the nail they do not migrate up the nail over time. Loss of the lunula reflects a low serum albumin and malnutrition.

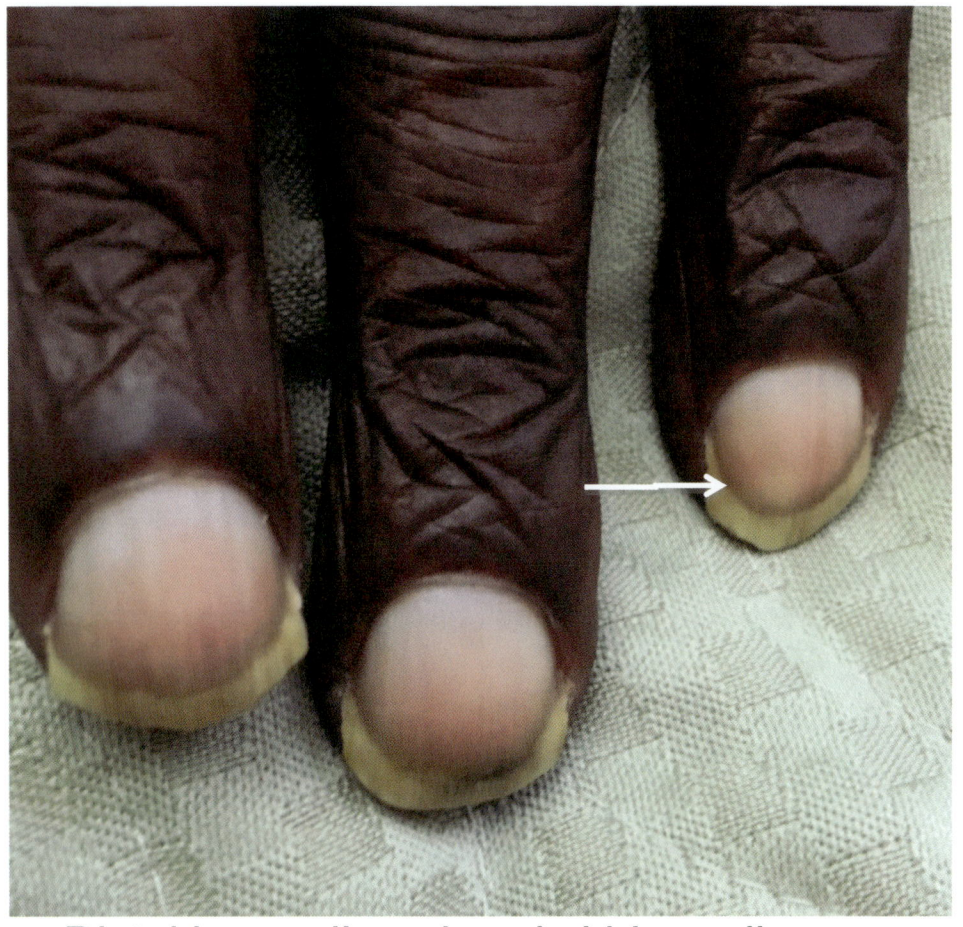

Distal brown line chronic kidney disease

TRANSVERSE DISTAL BROWN LINE

A transverse brown line just proximal to the free edge of the nail suggests chronic kidney disease. The mechanism of this change is not known. Note the nail pallor implying anemia and the downward curvature suggesting secondary hyperparathyroidism.

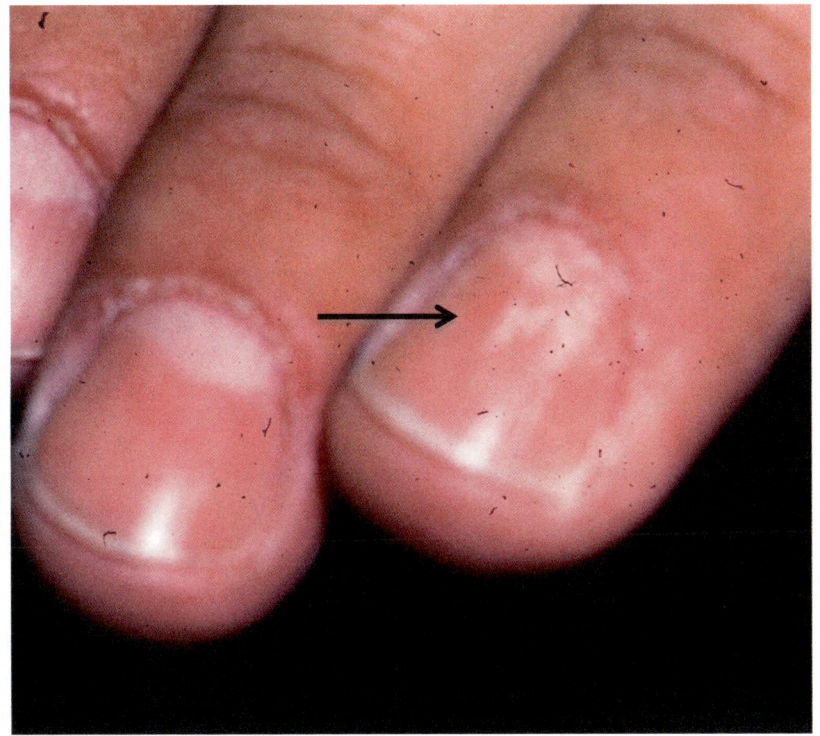

Leukonychia striae

WHITE CLOUD-LIKE SPLOTCHES

White cloud-like splotches are commonly seen on the nails. The medical term for them is leukonychia striae. They are caused by minor trauma to the nail matrix that allows immature nucleated cells to be incorporated into the nail. These nucleated cells give the nail a milky appearance. The timing of the trauma is inferred by the location of the "cloud" on the nail.

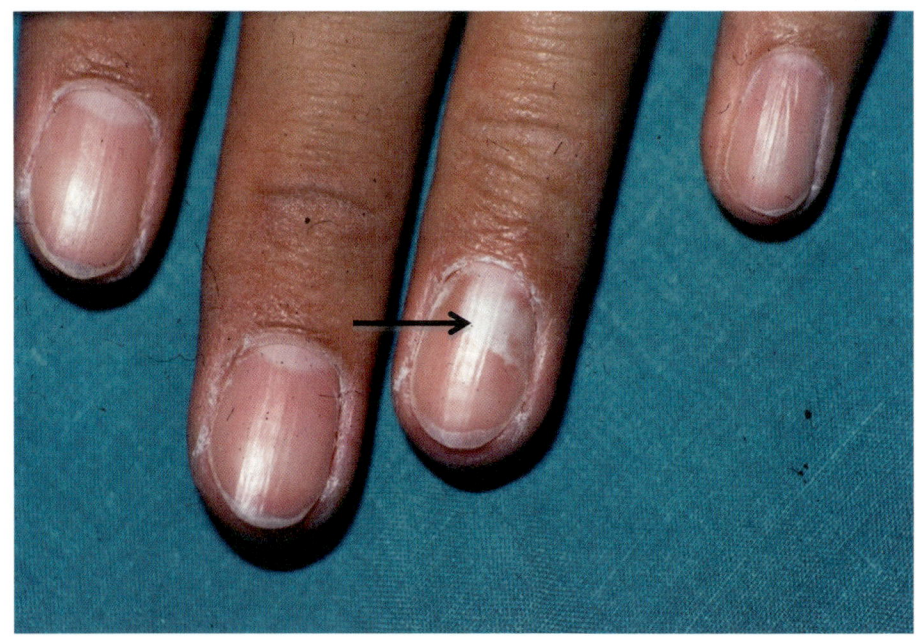

Proximal Onychomycosis

If the white discoloration is irregular and proximal with involvement of the cuticle consider proximal onychomycosis, an HIV defining condition. Notice the subtle redness behind the cuticle.

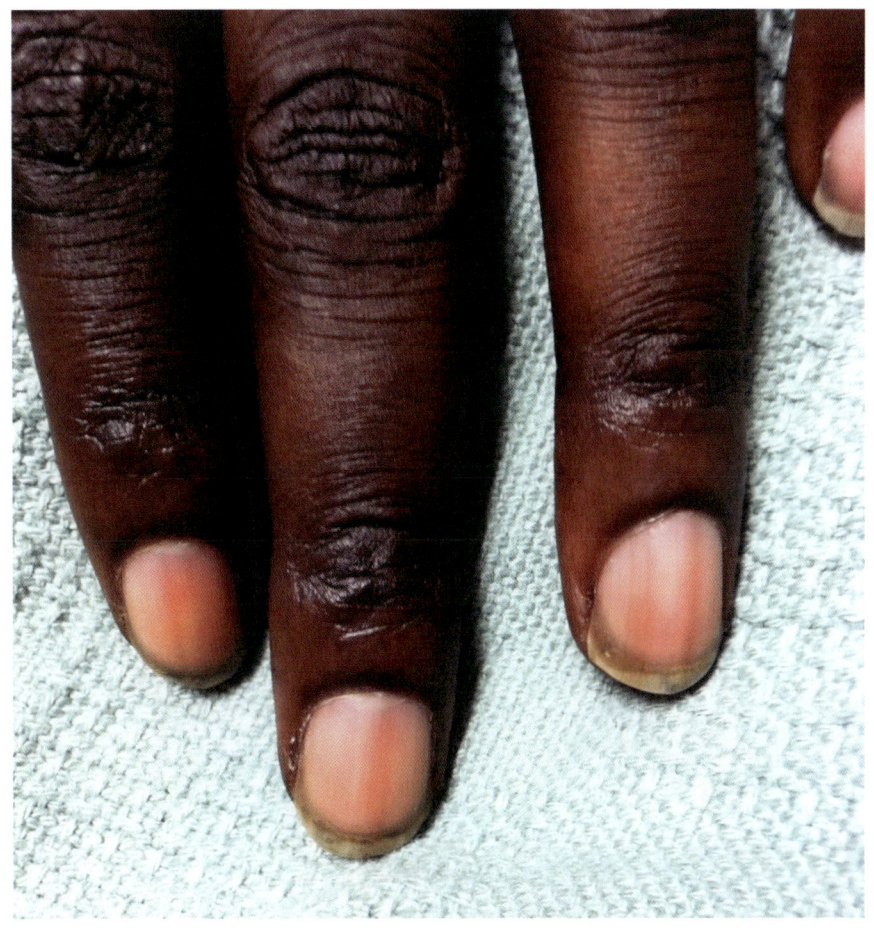

Longitudinal brown lines

LONGITUDINAL BROWN LINES

Longitudinal brown lines reflect increased melanin production by melanocytes in the nail matrix. When you see them, think of hyper-pigmenting conditions. These lines are associated with

Addison's disease, ectopic ACTH production, visible nevus at the nail base, breast cancer, melanoma (check for periungal pigmentation or destruction), trauma (especially for dark skinned individuals), and drugs.

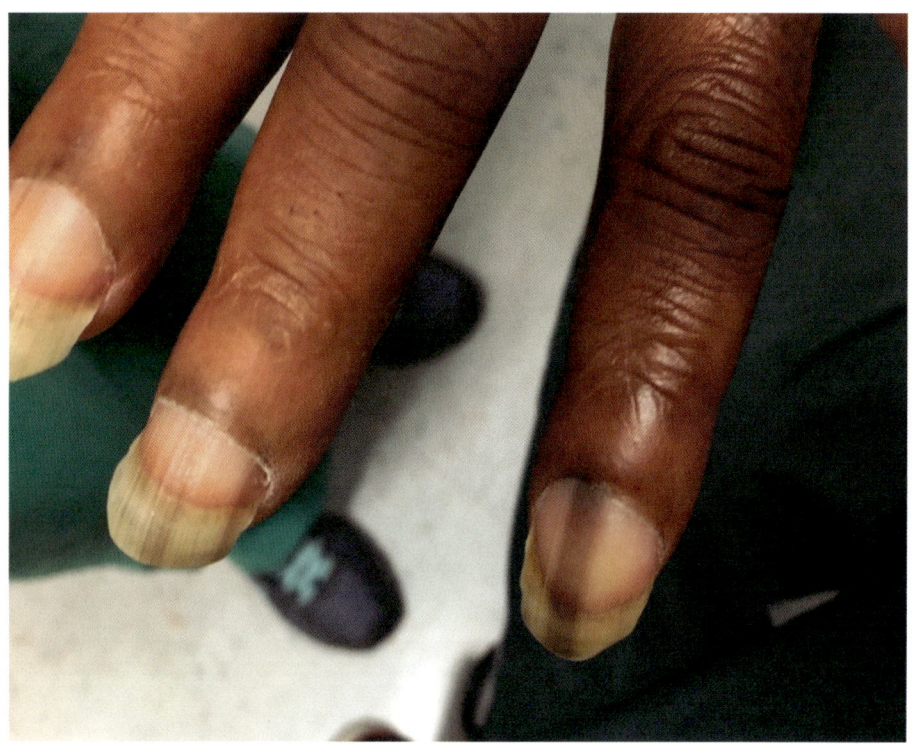

Traumatic brown line (sharp edges)

The lines produced by trauma tend to be sharper with more distinct edges. Medications effects tend to darken the entire nail.

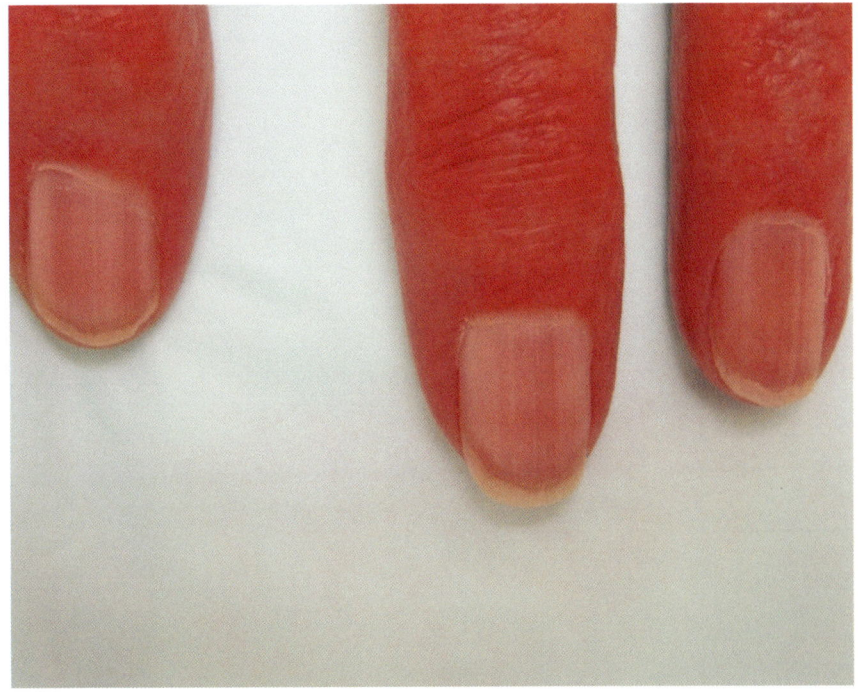

Longitudinal red lines

LONGITUDINAL RED LINES

Longitudinal pink or red lines are sometimes called "Heller's" lines or "candy cane nails." They suggest peripheral vascular disease particularly peripheral arterial disease.

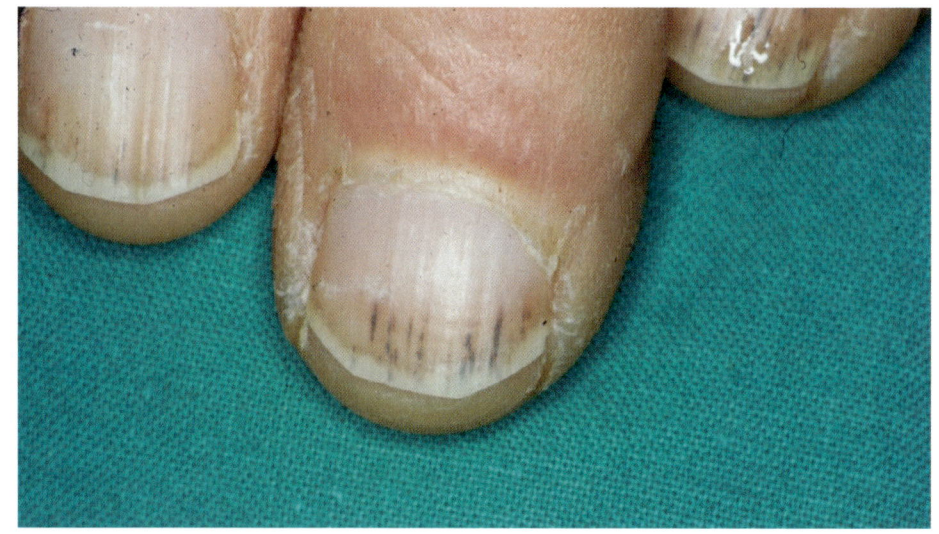

Splinter hemorrhages

SMALL BROWN LINES

Small brown or red longitudinal lines in the nail are called splinter hemorrhages, an important clue of infectious endocarditis. They should be differentiated from the black hair-like discolorations produced by trauma in that they are wider and fuller. The mechanism is hemorrhage of the distal capillary loops. In addition to infectious endocarditis, systemic lupus erythematosis, trichinosis (very exuberant splinters), pityriasis rubra pilaris can also cause splinter hemorrhages.

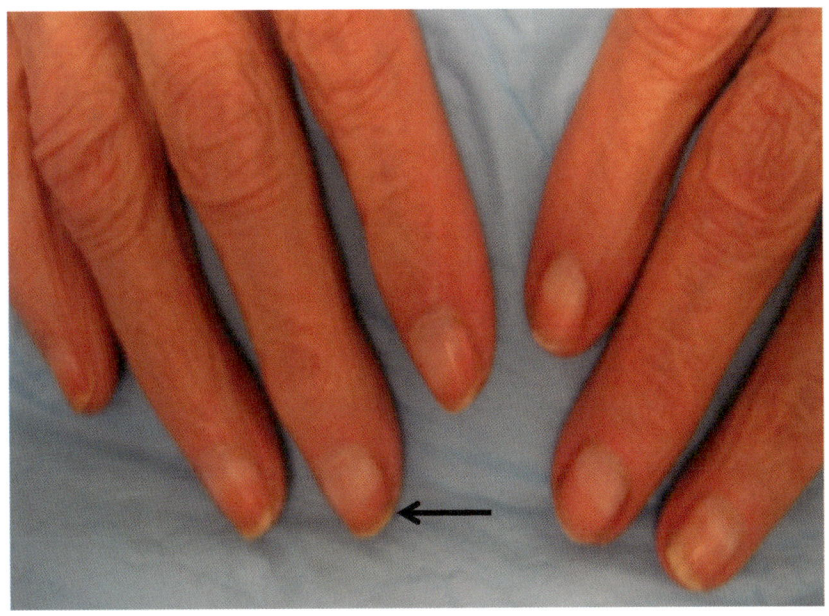

Terry's half-and-half nails from renal disease (with distal brown line)

TERRY'S HALF-AND-HALF NAILS

Terry's half-and-half nails are pale at the base and dark red at the free edge. If you can clearly see the lunula they are not Terry's nails. Imagine the following rhetorical inner dialogue: "Wow that is a large lunula. Wait a minute, <u>nothing makes the lunula larger</u>. So these must be Terry's half-and- half nails." Terry's half-and-half nails suggest chronic renal or liver disease.

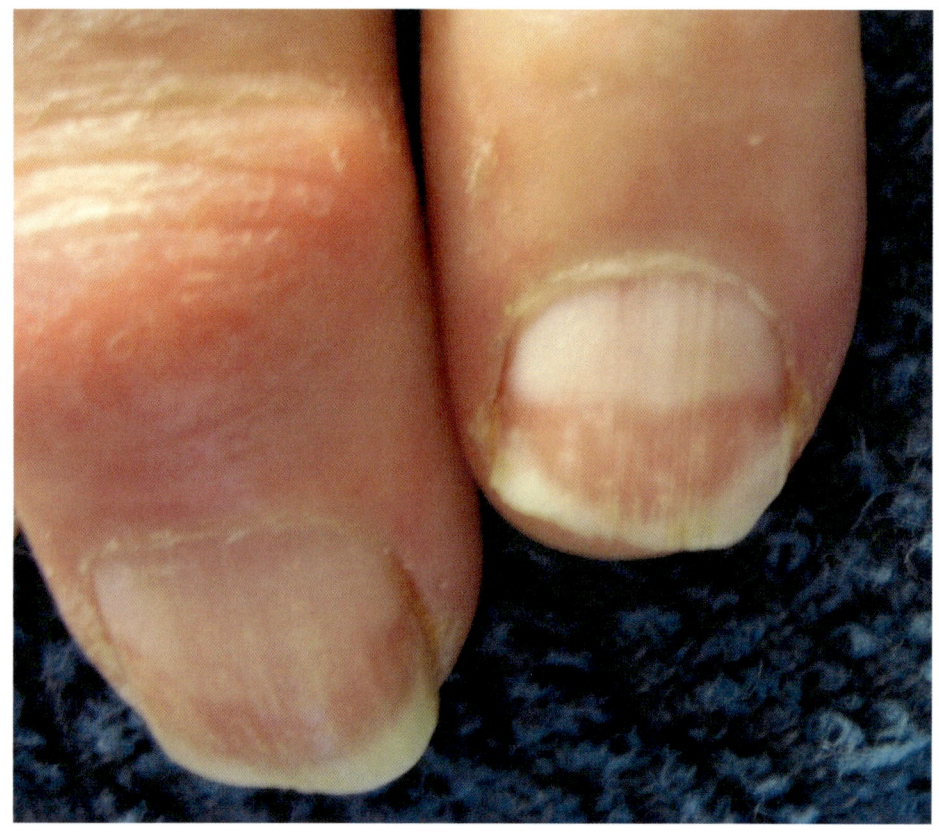

Terry's half-and-half nails in liver disease (no distal brown line)

And you can determine the cause at the bedside. If there is a rust color line at the free edge then consider renal disease as the cause; no brown discoloration suggests chronic liver disease (See images).

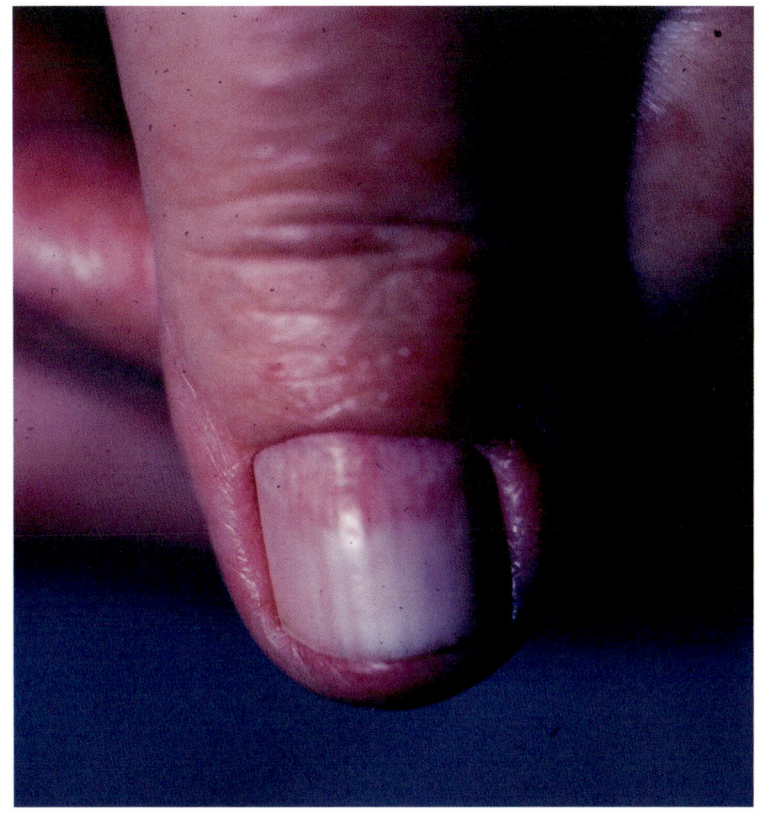

Terry's reversed half-and-half nail (red lunula)

Terry also described a half-and-half nail where the lunula and lower half of the nail is red and the upper half is pale. These nails (with a red lunula) suggest congestive heart failure, severe lung disease or hematological malignancy. These nails are covered in Chapter 2 on the lunula.

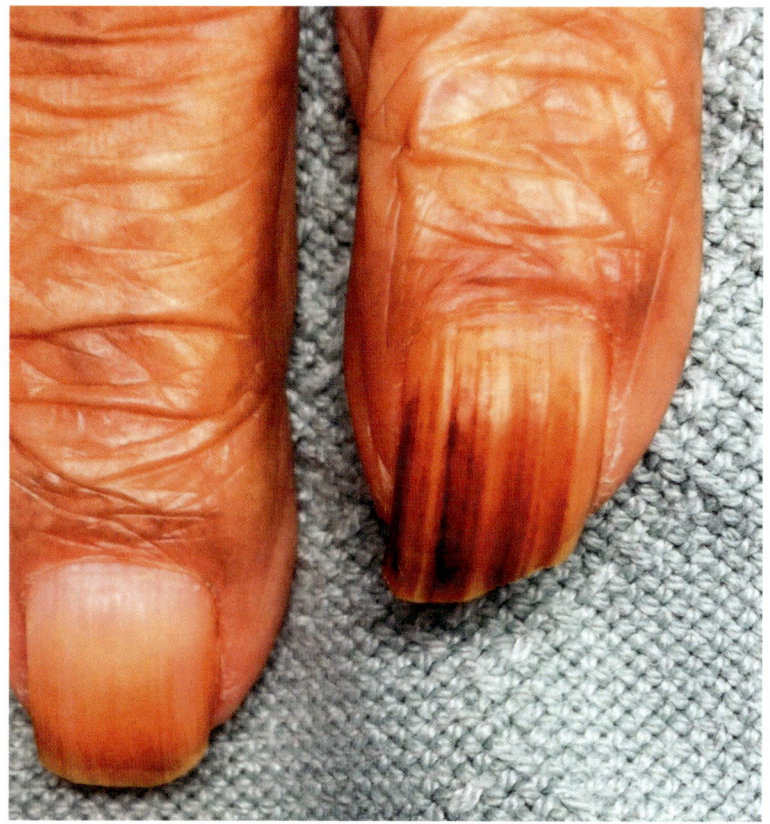

Yellow-brown nail from nicotine stain

NICOTINE STAIN

Nicotine can stain the nails a yellow-brown color. Characteristically is involves the index finger and middle finger to a lesser degree. This patient had stopped smoking a month ago. You might have inferred this because the base of the nail is much less stained.

Chapter 7

GENERALIZED NAIL DISCOLORATIONS

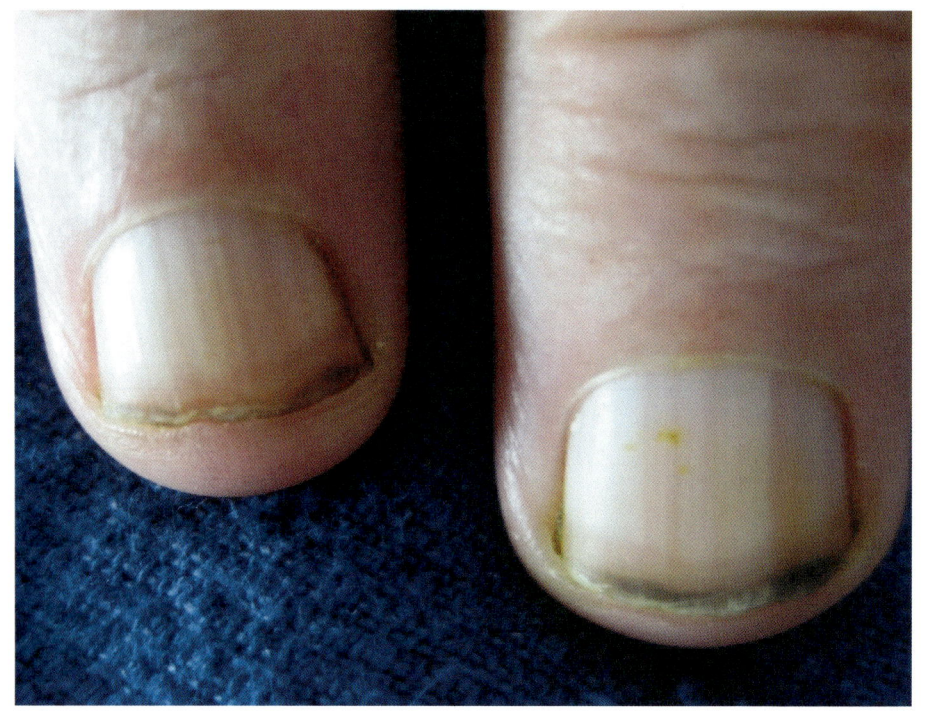

White nails

WHITE NAILS

These pale nails are caused by anemia, edema or vascular conditions. They resemble a Terry's half-and-half nail where the pallor has extended all the way to the free edge of the nail. Conditions to consider are anemia of any cause, chronic kidney disease (distal brown line at the free edge as in the image), chronic liver disease, and chemotherapy. There is also a rare hereditary white nail syndrome.

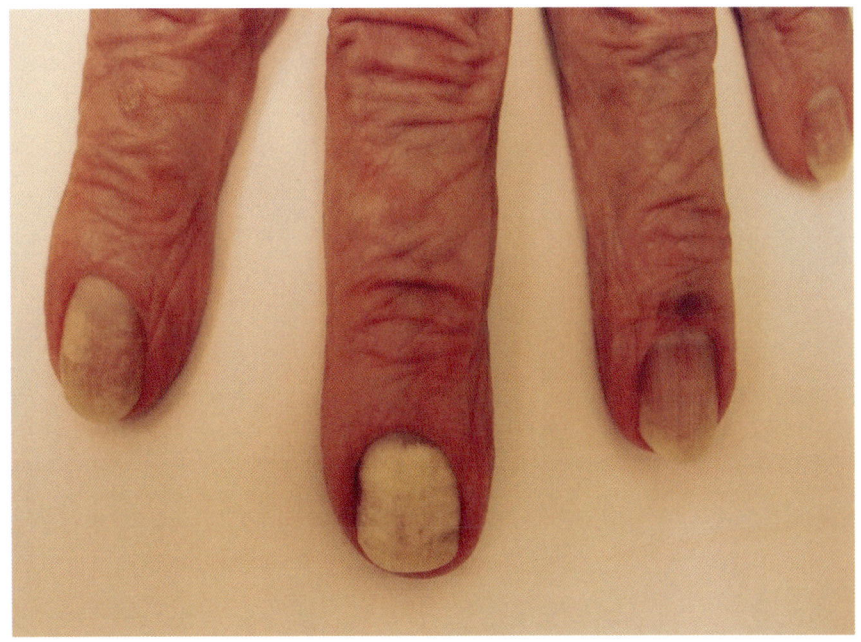

Local irregular white nails

LOCAL IRREGULAR WHITE NAILS

These nails suggest fungal disease called onychomycosis. As a useful rule of thumb, candida tends to affect the upper extremity nails while dermatophytes affect the toenails. As mentioned previously, proximal onychomycosis suggests HIV infection.

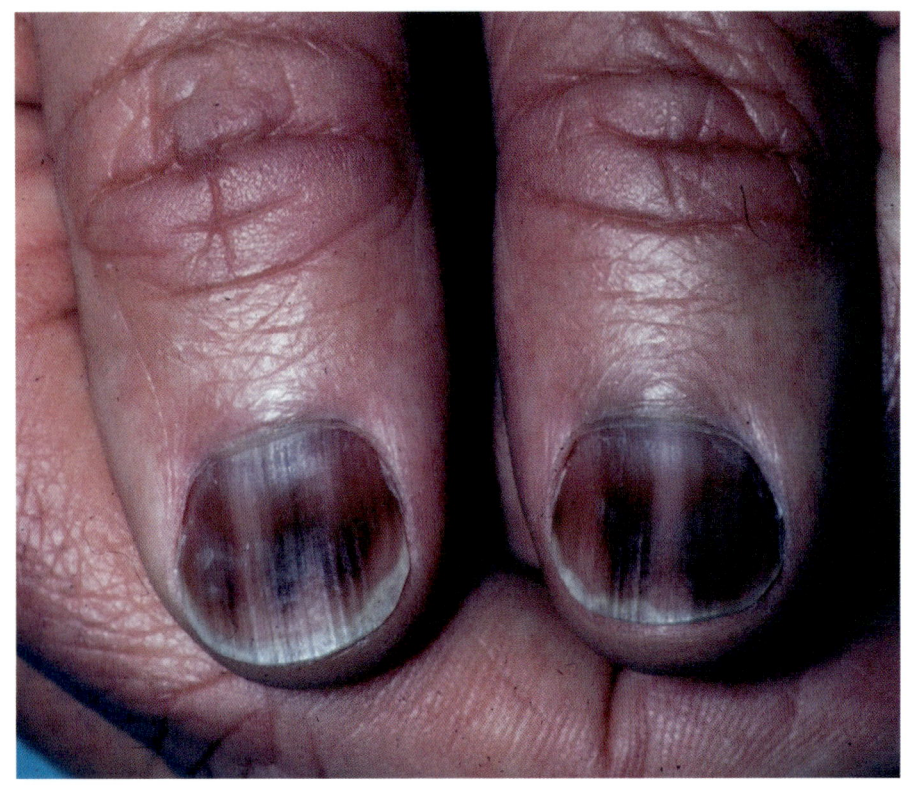

Brown nails

BROWN NAILS

Brown fingernails resemble nails stained with shoe polish. These suggest hyperpigmenting disorders such as vitamin B12 deficiency, Addison's disease, breast cancer, malignant melanoma, lichen planus, syphilis, topical agents, and drugs. AZT as part of HIV therapy can turn the nails brown and a long duration of therapy can darken the tone.

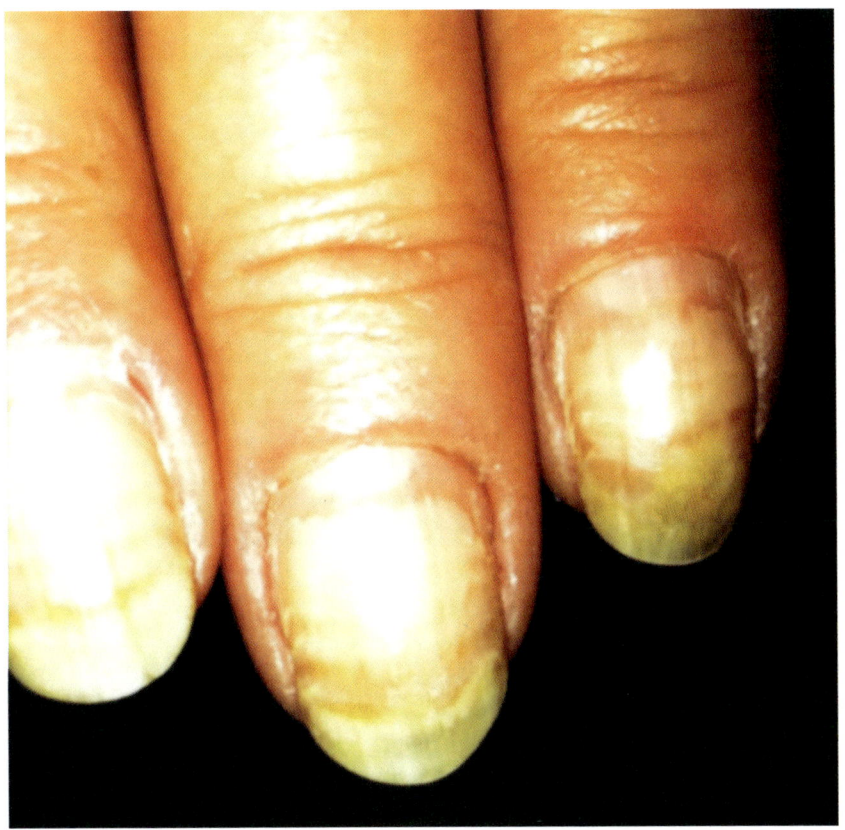

Yellow nails

YELLOW NAILS

When you see yellow nails think of diabetes mellitus. Yellow nails suggest lymphatic obstruction. Conditions other than diabetes mellitus to consider are peripheral nerve injury (yellowing in the nerve distribution), thermal injury, jaundice, systemic amyloidosis (very waxy and friable), and yellow nail syndrome.

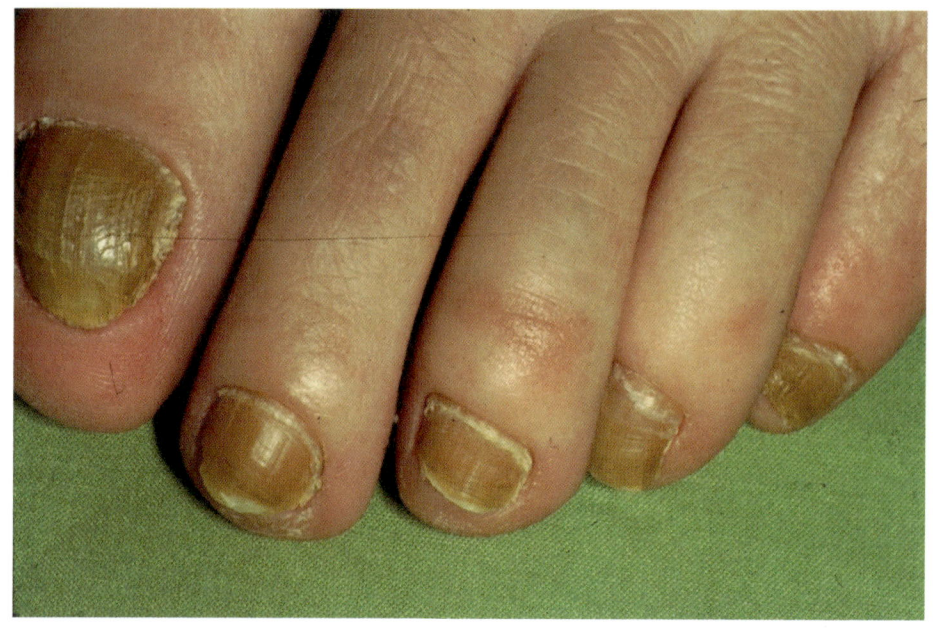

Yellow Nail Syndrome

Yellow nail syndrome is the triad of lymphedema, bronchiectasis, and bronze, brown colored nails (See Image).

GREEN OR BLACK NAILS

Green or black discolorations can result from topical preparations, chronic pseudomonas infection, toxic ingestion and trauma. The photo shows an example of pseudomonas infection treated for the last three months. You can infer the treatment period because the normal nail has grown out about halfway.

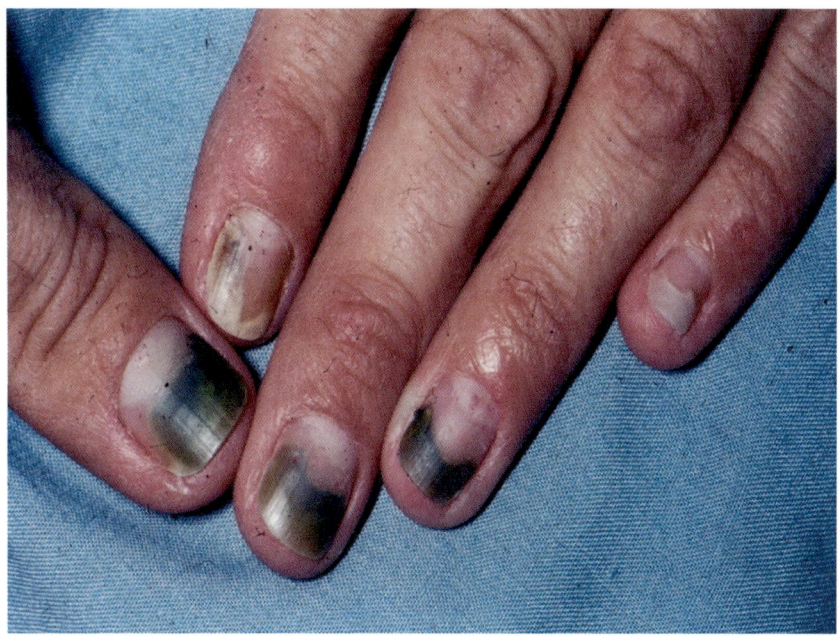

Green nails due to pseudomonas infection

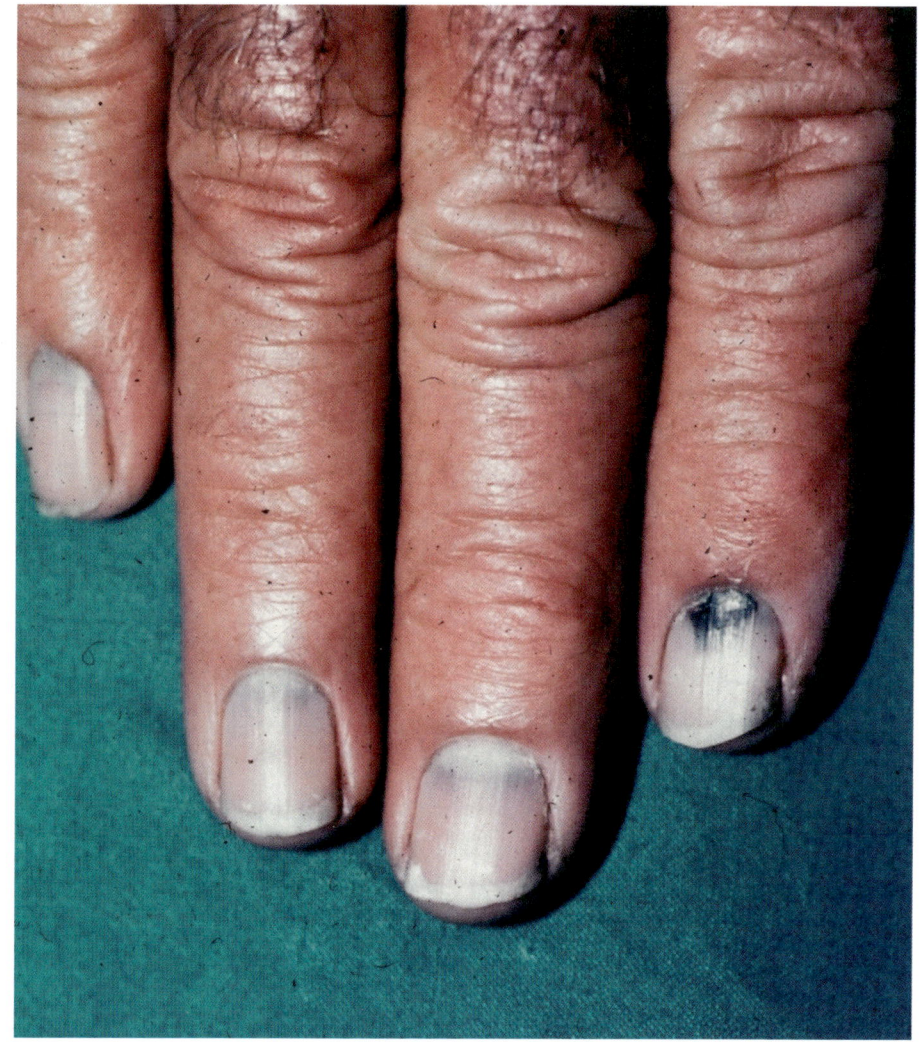

Black nails from Argyria]

Heavy metal toxicity can cause black nail pigmentation. This case of argyria was due to ingestion of colloidal silver salts over a two-month period as an alternative medicine remedy.

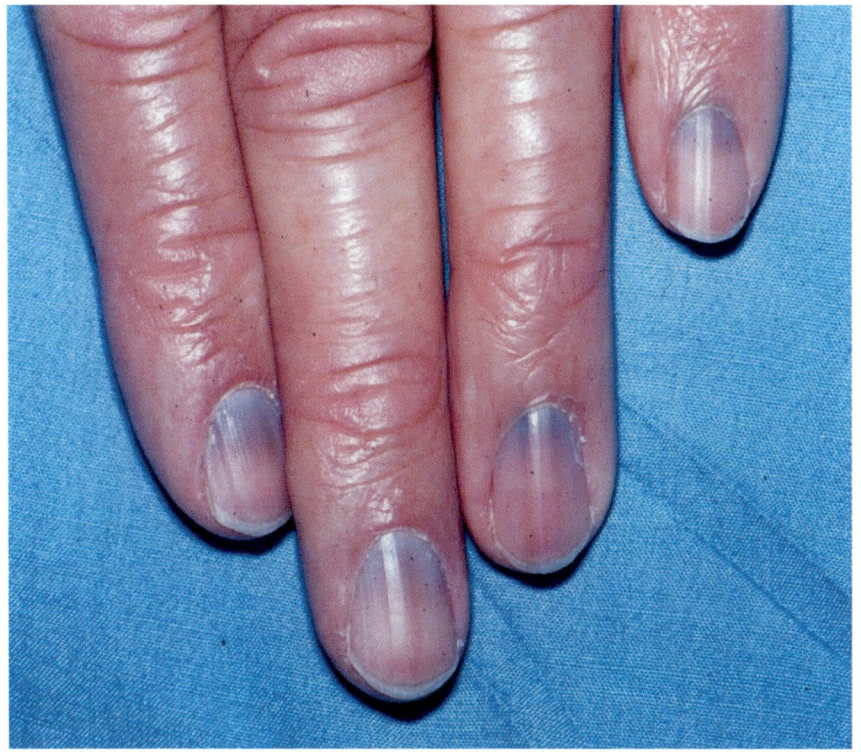

Blue nails from Minocycline

BLUE NAILS

Blue nails can obviously be seen in cyanosis. Another cause shown in the photo is minocycline ingestion. Generally more than 100 grams (cumulatively) of minocycline have to be ingested to increase the risk of this rare complication.

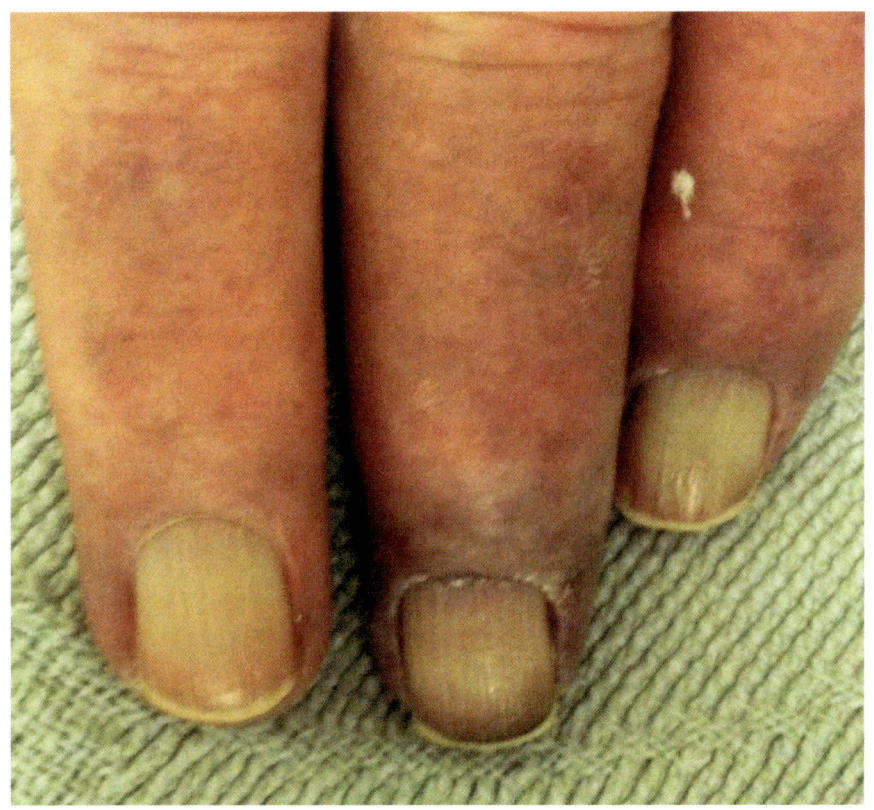

Purple nail from Raynaud's phenomenon

PURPLE NAILS

Cyanosis from any cause can produce a purple nail. In the image, the middle nail is purple from Raynaud's phenomenon. Also notice the loss of fine transverse wrinkles in the distal parts of the fingers suggesting systemic sclerosis.

Chapter 8

Processes Around the Nail

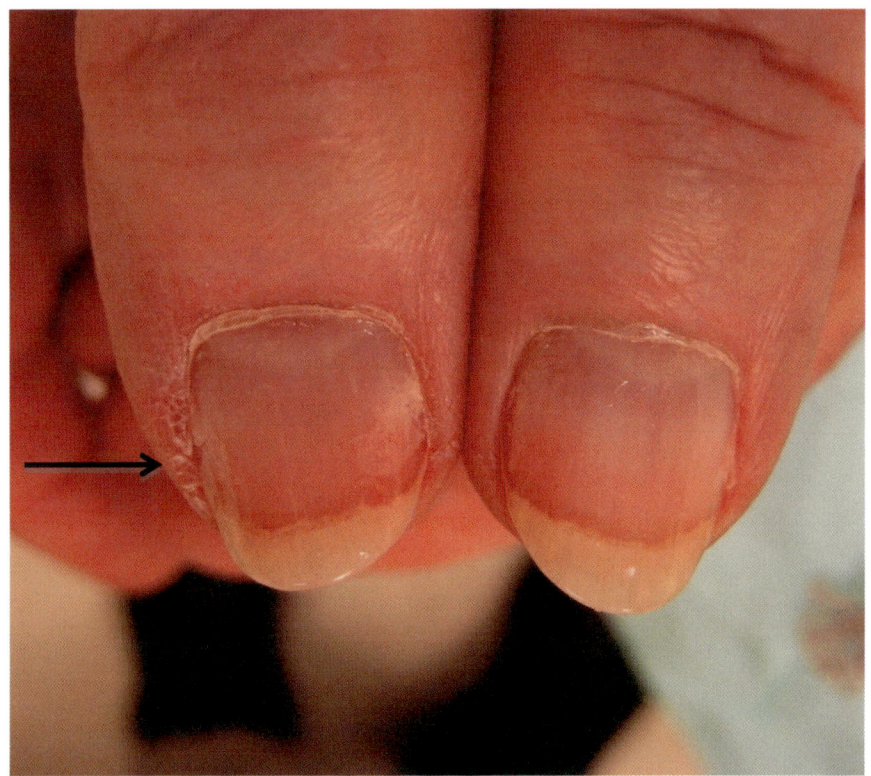

Paronychia

PARONYCHIA

Paronychias are common and result from infection along the edge of the nail. In chronic paronychial inflammation there is swelling, scaling and nail separation (onycholysis). Water exposure is a risk factor. Paronychias suggest stress, trauma, bacterial infection, or herpetic whitlow. Healing can produce deformity along the side of the nail. Pseudomonas paronychia can turn the nail green.

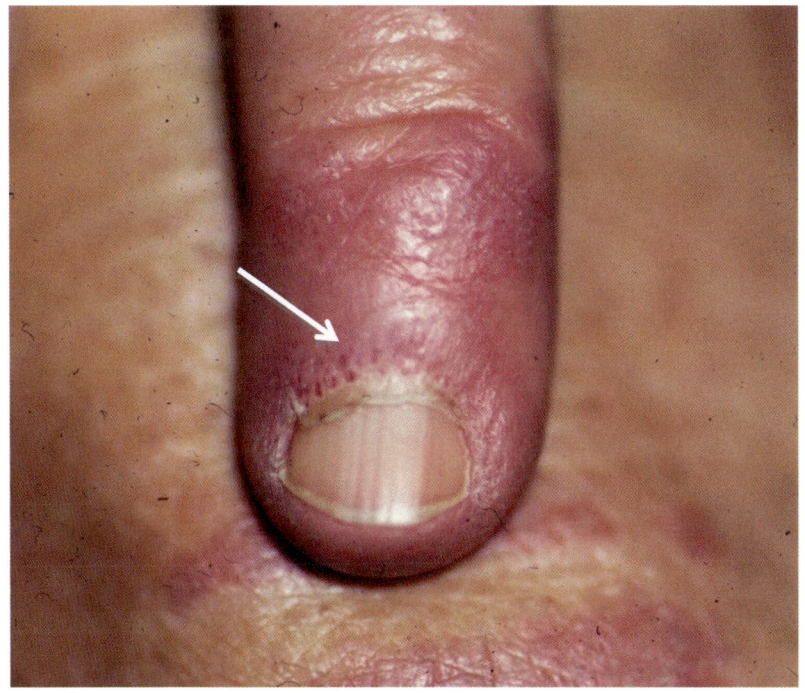

Dilated capillary loops

DILATED CAPILLARY LOOPS

Seeing dilated capillary loops is a very important observation because the findings are associated with autoimmune conditions that are sometimes tricky to diagnose. The key features are atrophy of the cuticle and the presence of dilated capillary loops called periungal telangiectasia. They <u>strongly</u> associated with systemic lupus erythemayosis, dermatomyositis, systemic sclerosis, and vasculitis.

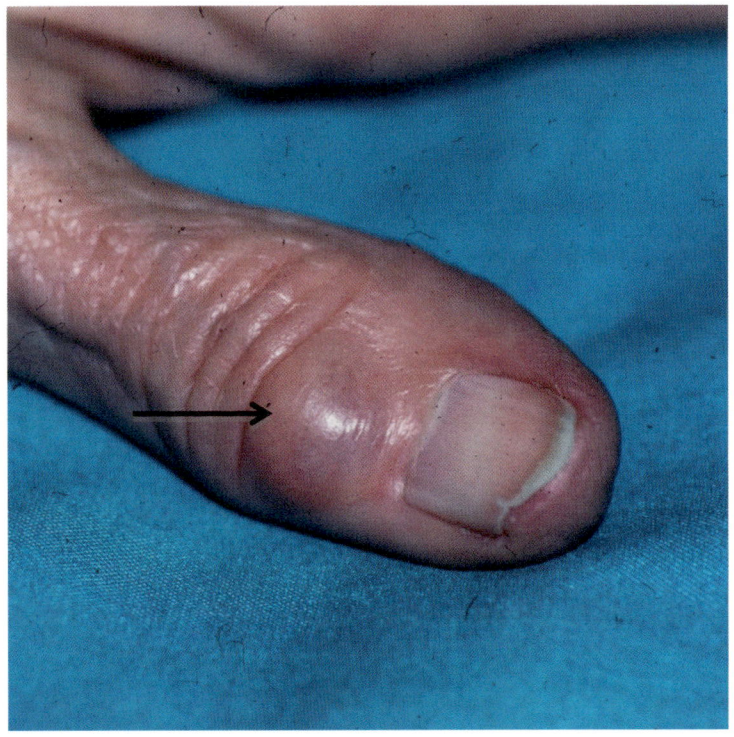

Mucus cyst

MUCUS CYST

A mucus cyst is a painless fluid filled swelling that occurs most commonly at the proximal interphalangeal joint. They are associated with osteoarthritis. The cyst sits anatomically above the matrix and pushes down on it creating a gutter along the nail distal to the cyst. They are benign and may disappear over time.

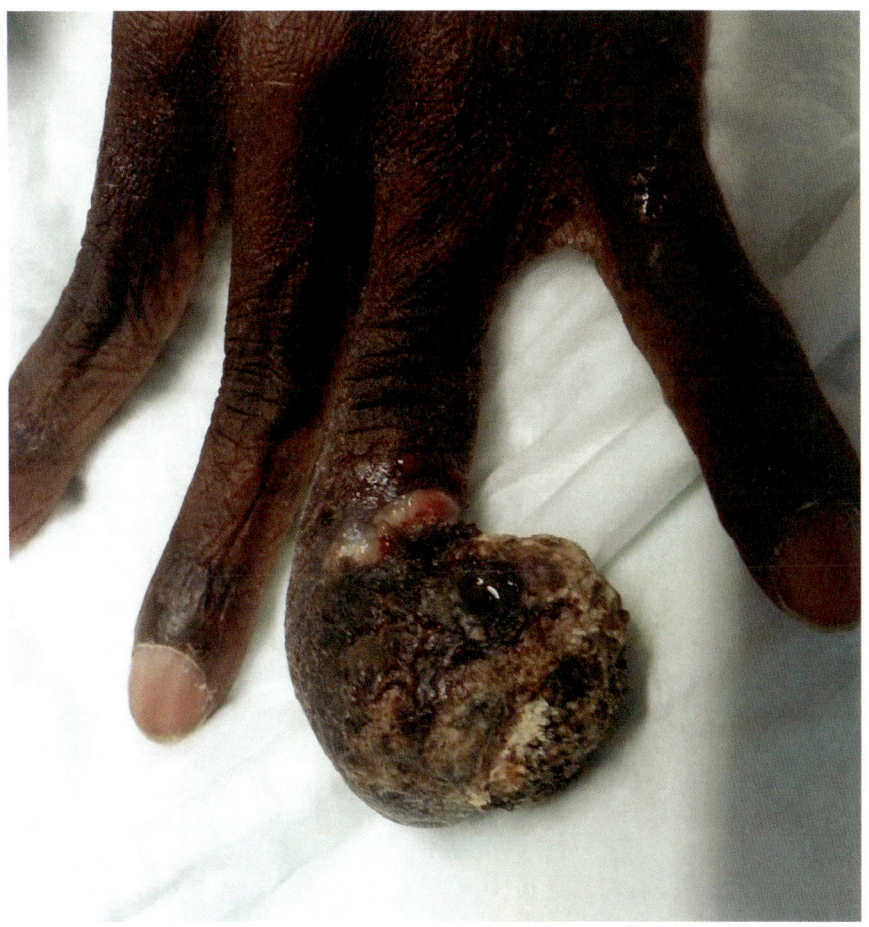

Pyogenic granuloma from blastomycosis

A pyogenic granuloma is neither pus producing (pyogenic) nor a granuloma. It is a capillary hemangioma that exhibits "proud flesh." Pyogenic granuloma can grow rapidly and are likely to bleed. They are sometimes related to trauma. This remarkable image shows the reaction to blastomycosis in a person with HIV.

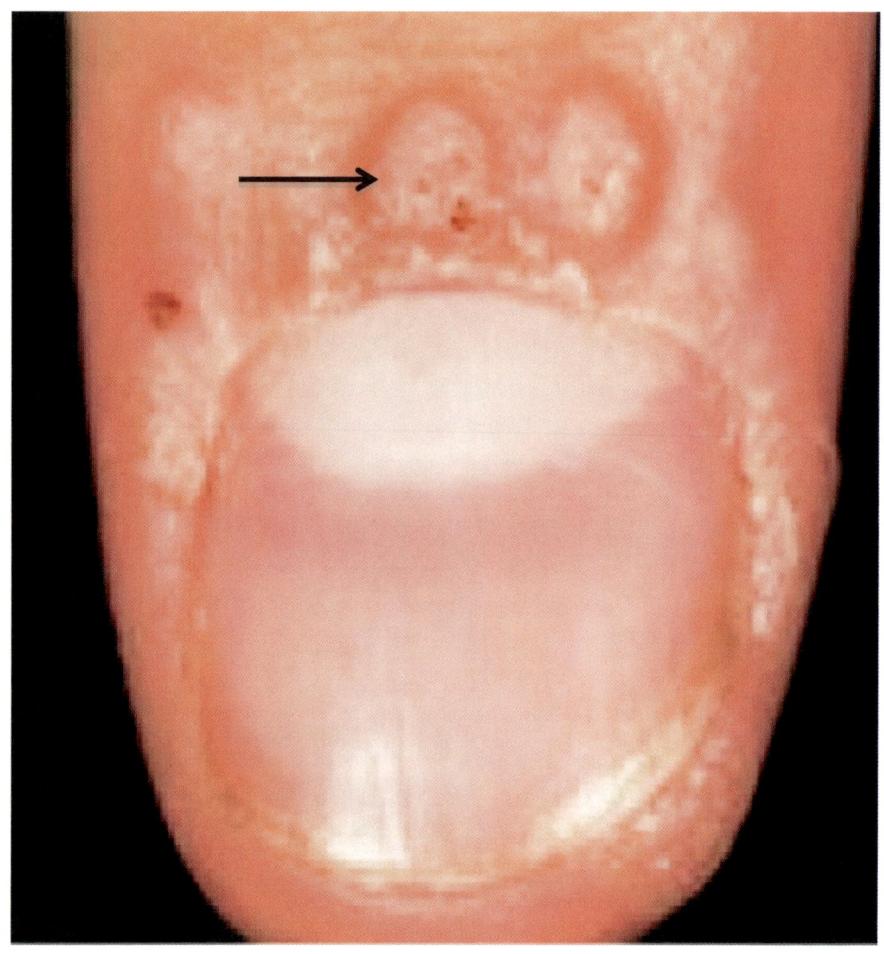

Warts

Warts are caused by human papilloma virus and are easily identifiable by the raised dome shaped rough surface.

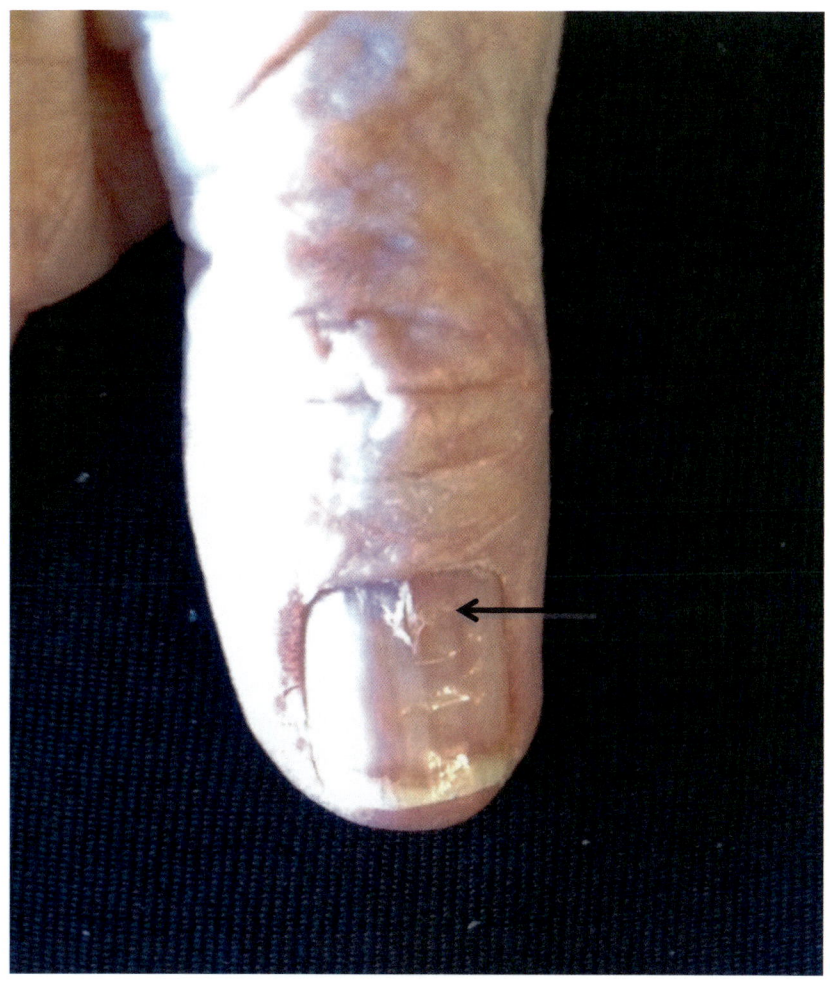

Fibrokeratoma

A fibrokeratoma is a pink pointed painless mass that lifts off the nail. It is benign and composed of connective tissue. It tends to grow slowly and distort the nail plate.

Chapter 9

Case Presentations

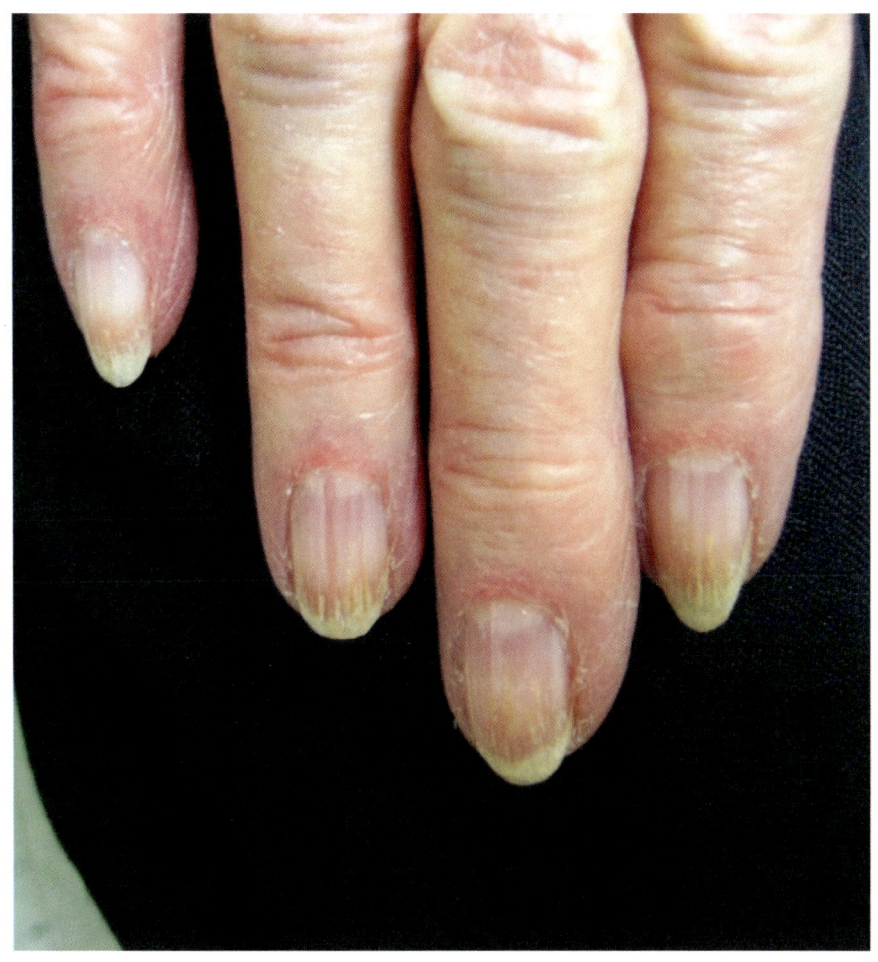

Case 1

Case 1

A 73-year-old woman presents with fatigue and loss of vitality.

What conditions do her fingernails suggest?

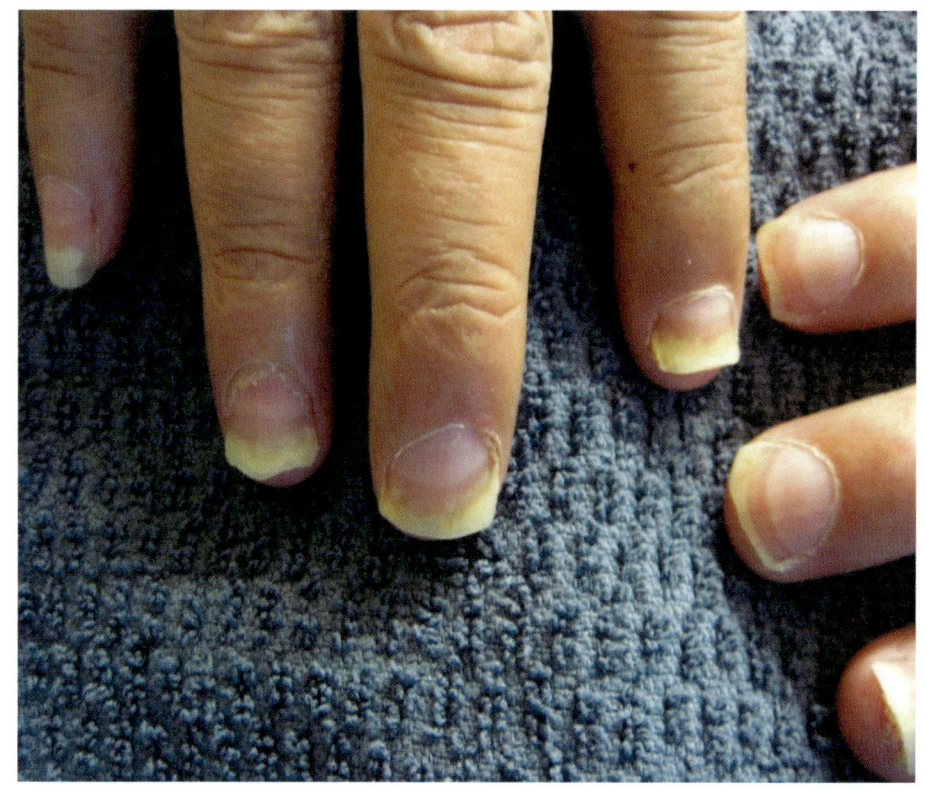

Case 2

Case 2

A 52-year-old woman is seen in your clinic for peripheral edema and abdominal swelling. What illness would most likely produce these nails?

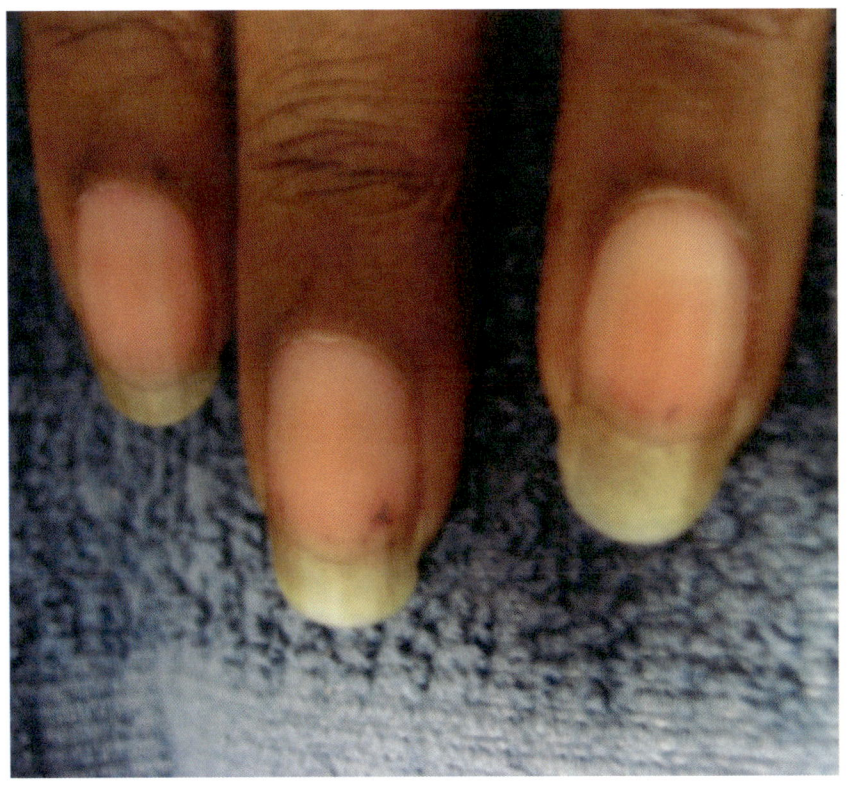

Case 3

Case 3

You see a 57 year-old-woman with fever, malaise, and muscle aches.

In addition to infectious endocarditis what condition is most likely to produce these nail findings?

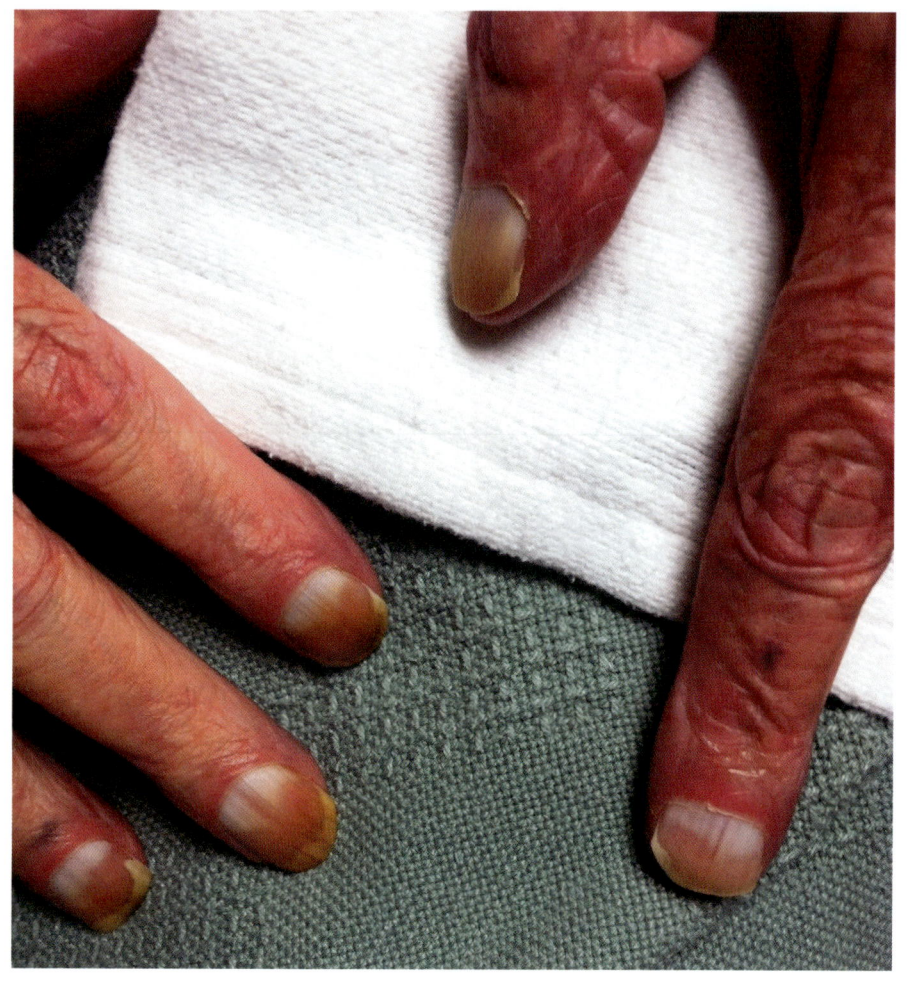

Case 4

Case 4

A 71-year-old man presents with lethargy, fatigue and anorexia. What is your diagnosis and the fingernail evidence that supports it?

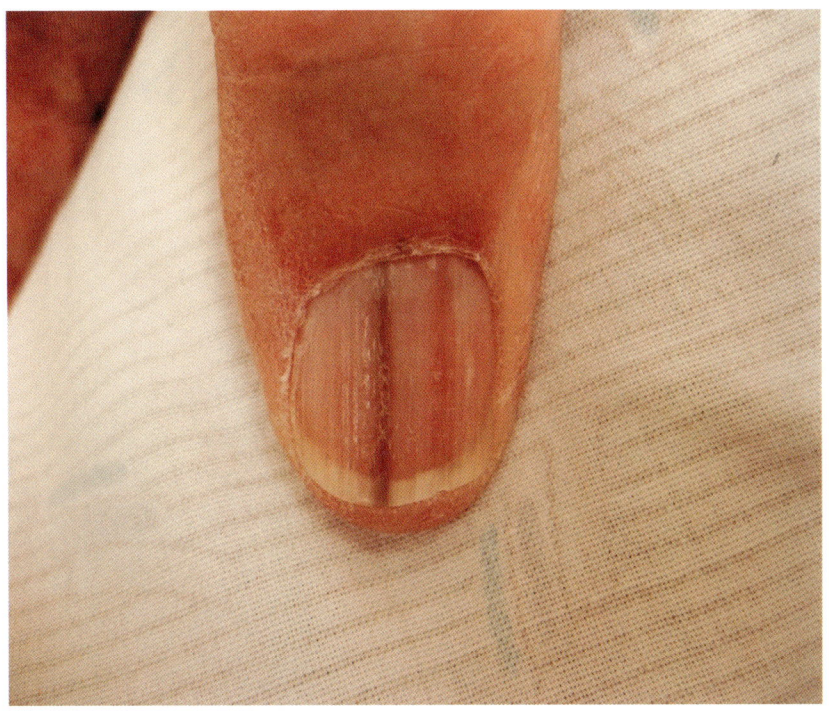

Case 5

Case 5

A 66-year-old man visits your clinic with complaints of fatigue, hypotension and an increased sense of smell. There is no history of finger trauma. What conditions are suggested from his thumbnail?

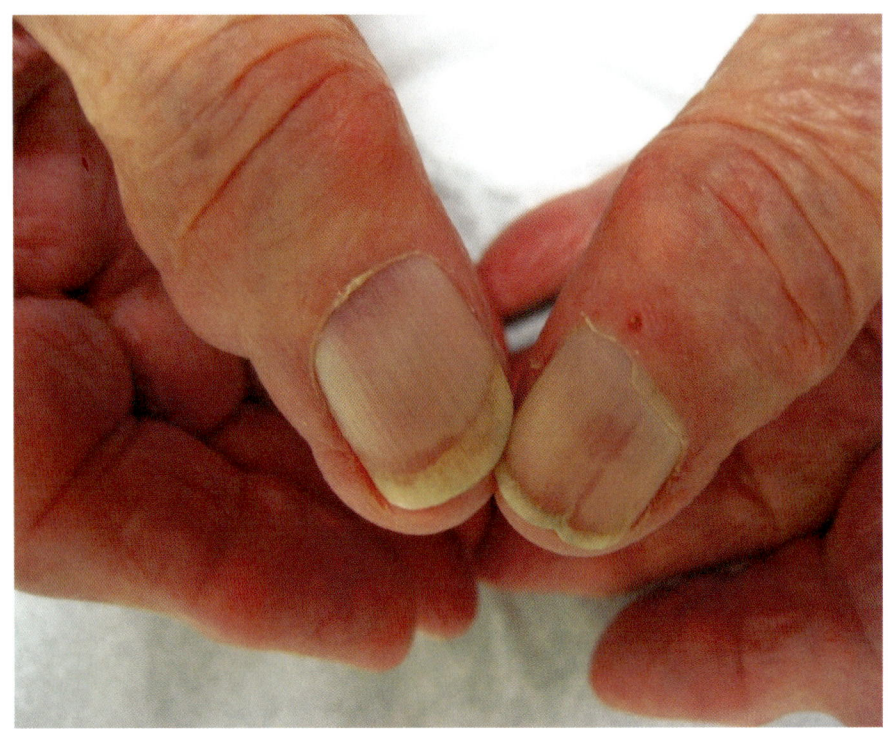

Case 6

Case 6

An 84 year old man sees you in your clinic for a painful ankle.

Name five likely diseases on his problem list.

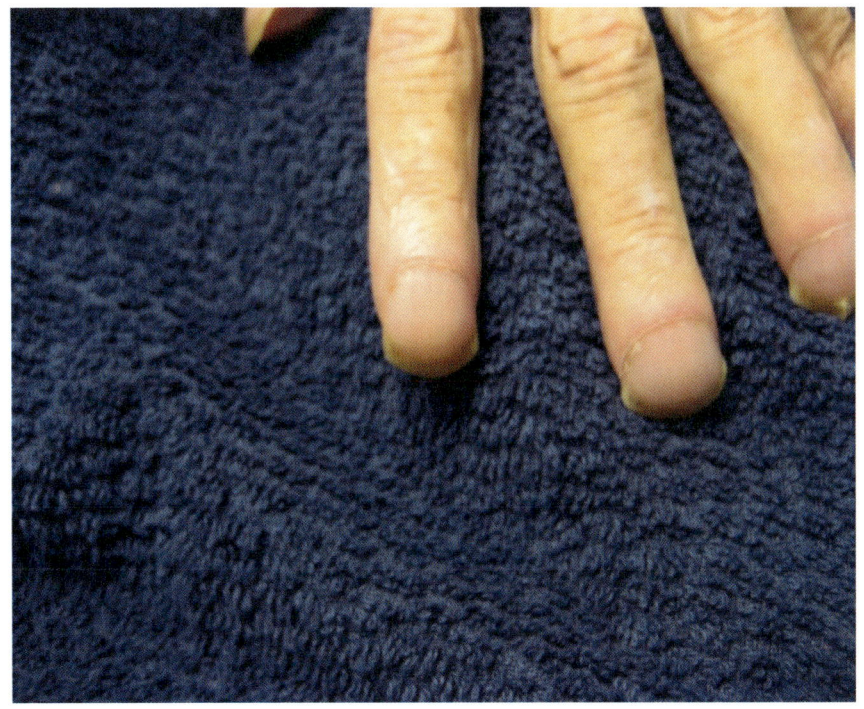

Case 7

Case 7

A 68-year-old man presents with weight loss and dysphagia. You examine his hands and suspect a specific diagnosis.

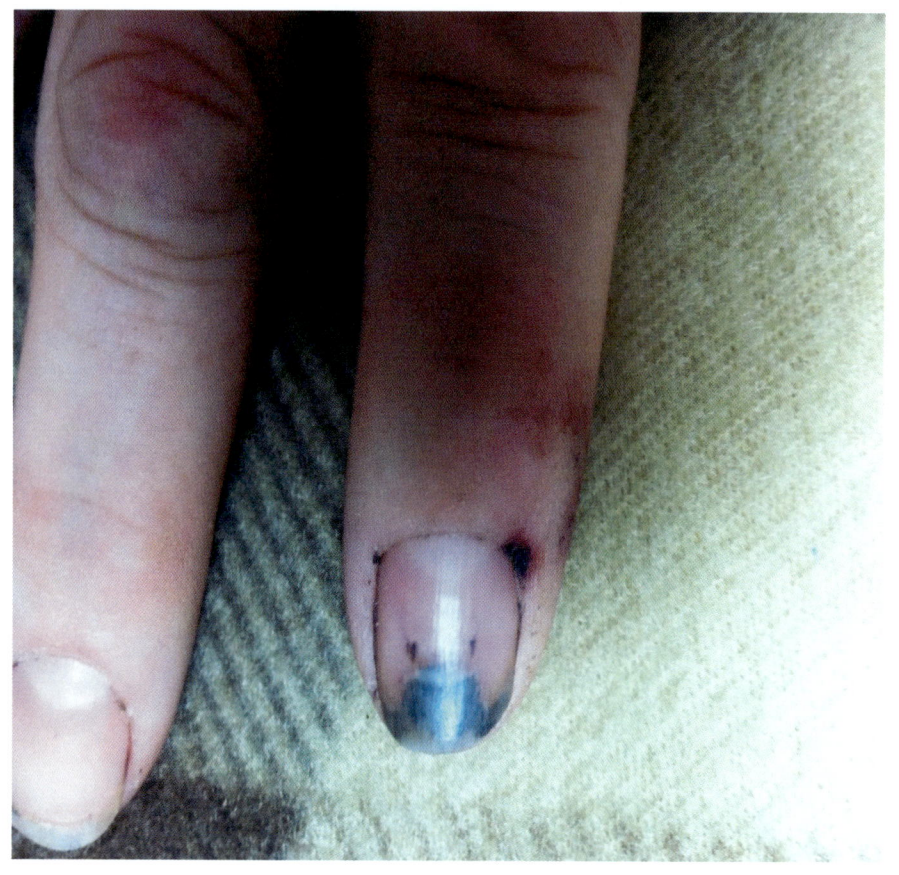

Case 8

Case 8

A 62 year old woman presents with fever, malaise, proximal muscle weakness, dysphagia, vague lower abdominal pain and weight loss. There is a rash over the skin between the knuckles. What is the most likely diagnosis?

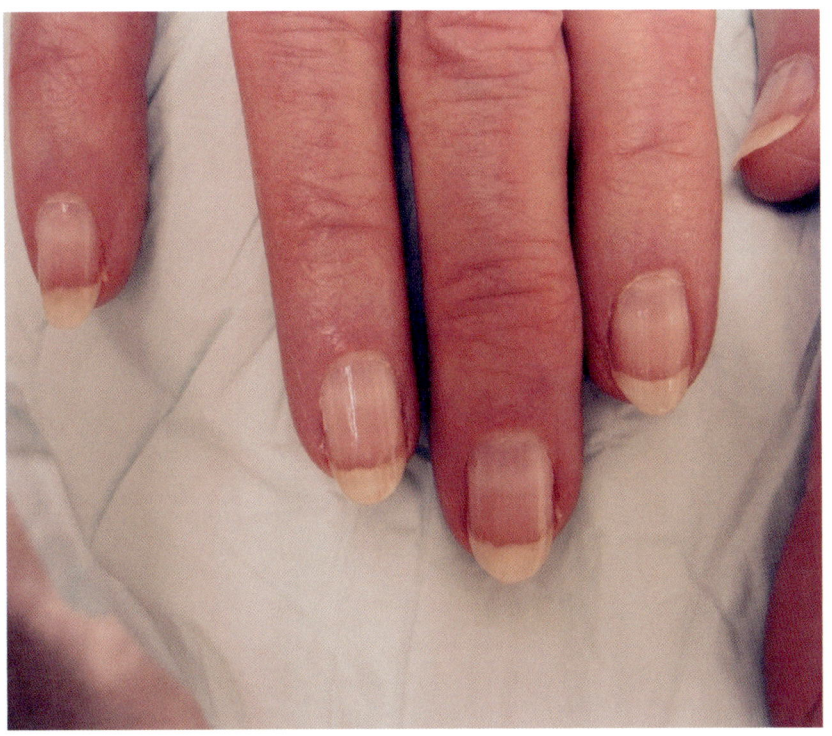

Case 9

Case 9

A 73-year-old woman presents to your clinic for a new patient evaluation. What can you infer about her clinical condition from her nails?

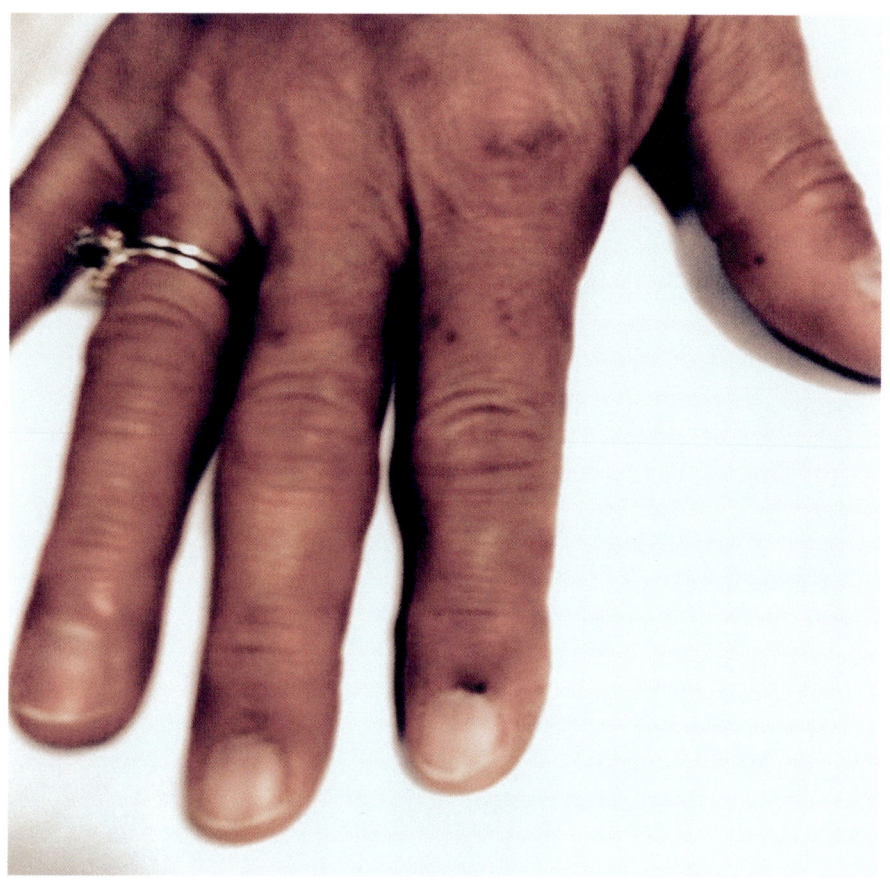

Case 10

Case 10

A 55-year-old woman presents with fever, fatigue, muscle pain and pleuritic chest pain. What is the most likely diagnosis?

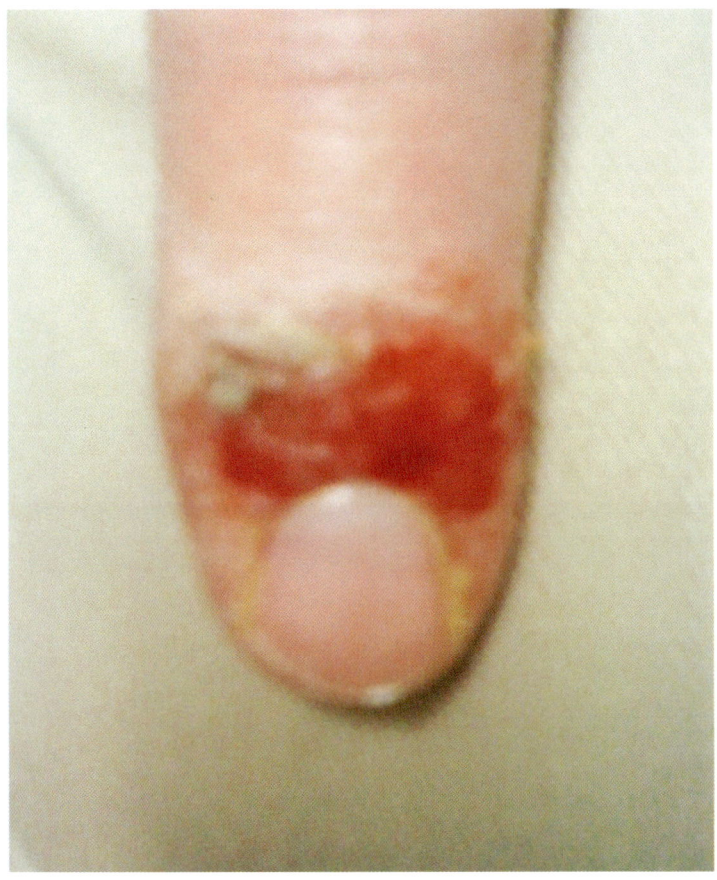

Case 11

Case 11

A 70-year-old man comes to your office complaining of a painful forefinger. The redness began two weeks ago with swelling at the base of the nail. He has noticed some purulent drainage. What is the most likely explanation for the process?

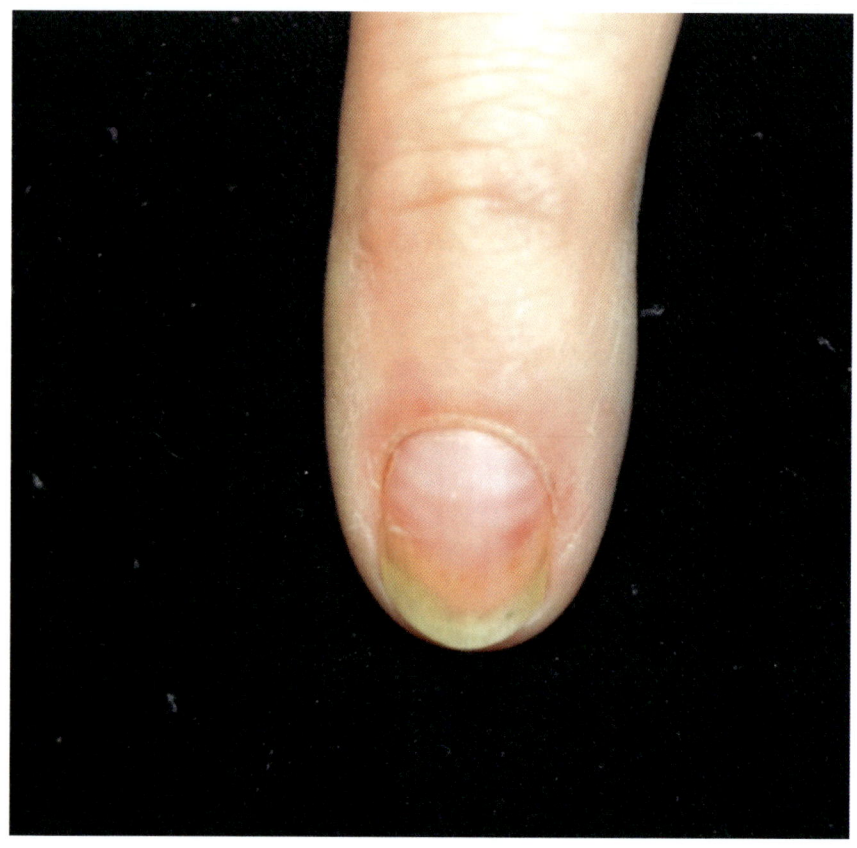

Case 12

Case 12

A 54-year-old woman comes to your clinic for an initial visit. What can you infer about her medical history from her fingernails?

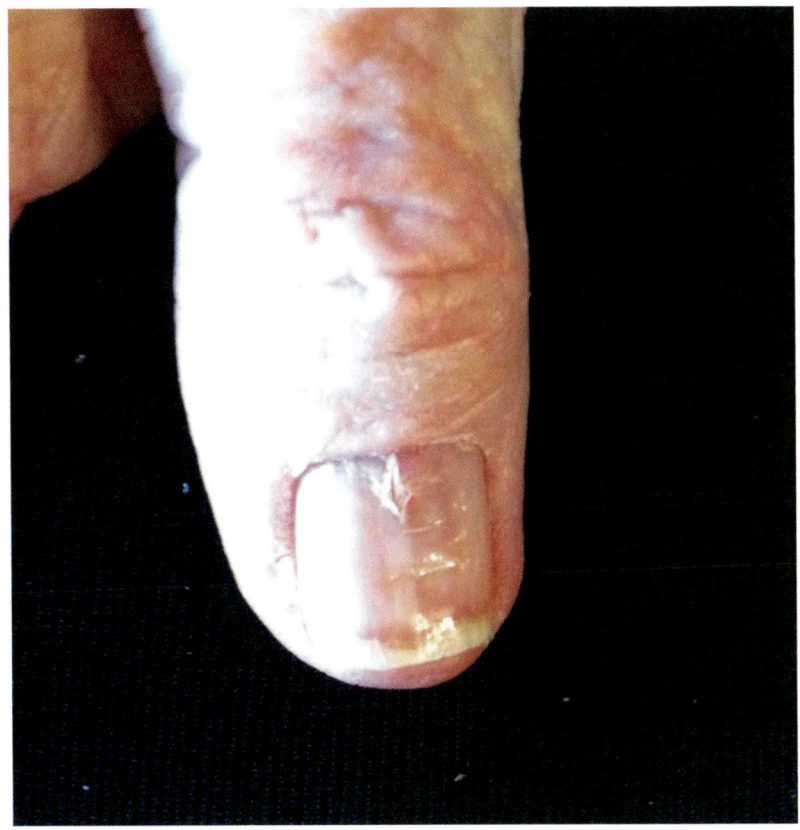

Case 13

Case 13

An 80-year-old woman has noticed a growth on her thumbnail. It started as a painless, fleshy pink, firm mass. It feels firm and has remained in place for the past four months. There is no history of trauma. None of her other nails are affected. What is the most likely diagnosis of her condition?

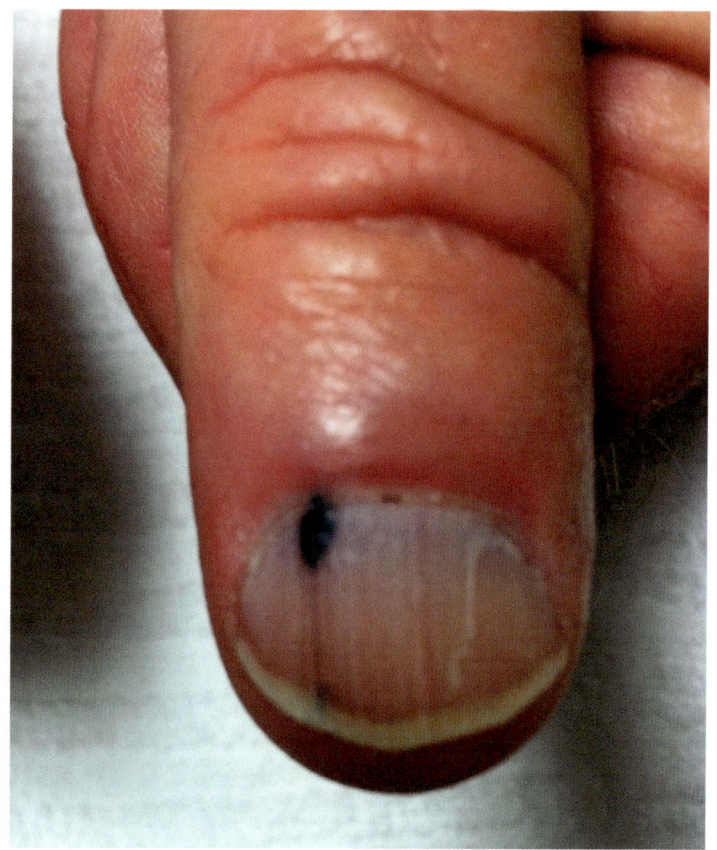

Case 14

Case 14

A 78-year-old man tells you that he is beginning a new relationship and would like to know what is causing this new painless discoloration of his thumb. There is no history of trauma. What is the most likely reason for his nail findings?

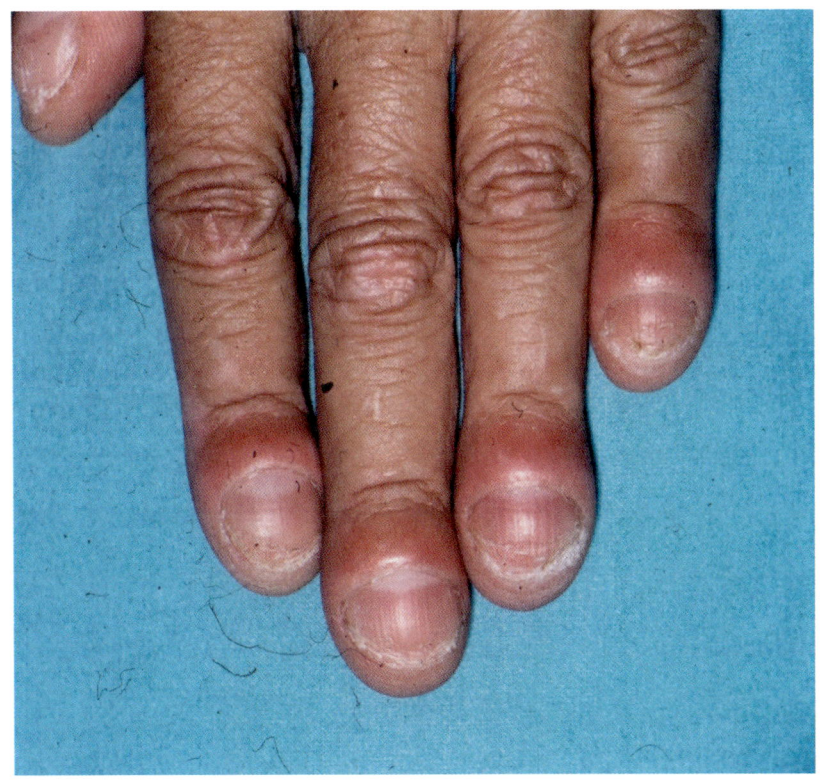

Case 15

Case 15

A 61-year-old man presents with persistent non-productive cough, fatigue and an involuntary twenty-pound weight loss over the past four months. He has no GI complaints. What serious diagnosis should you consider?

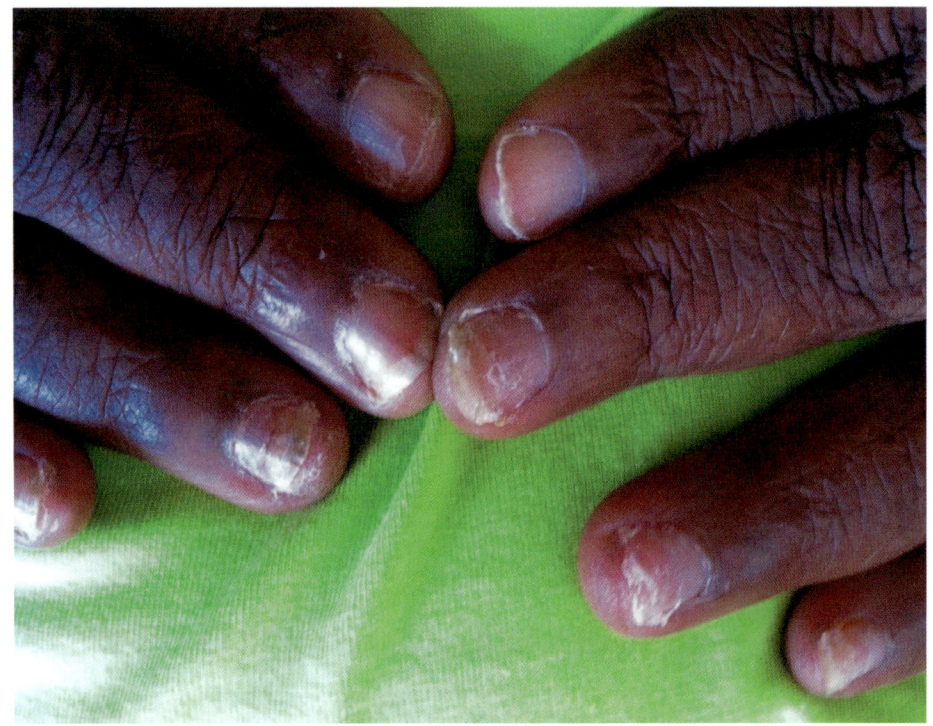

Case 16

Case 16

A 59-year-old woman has been on antifungal treatment following a bone marrow transplant and infection with invasive aspergillosis. What antifungal treatment is most likely to cause these nail changes?

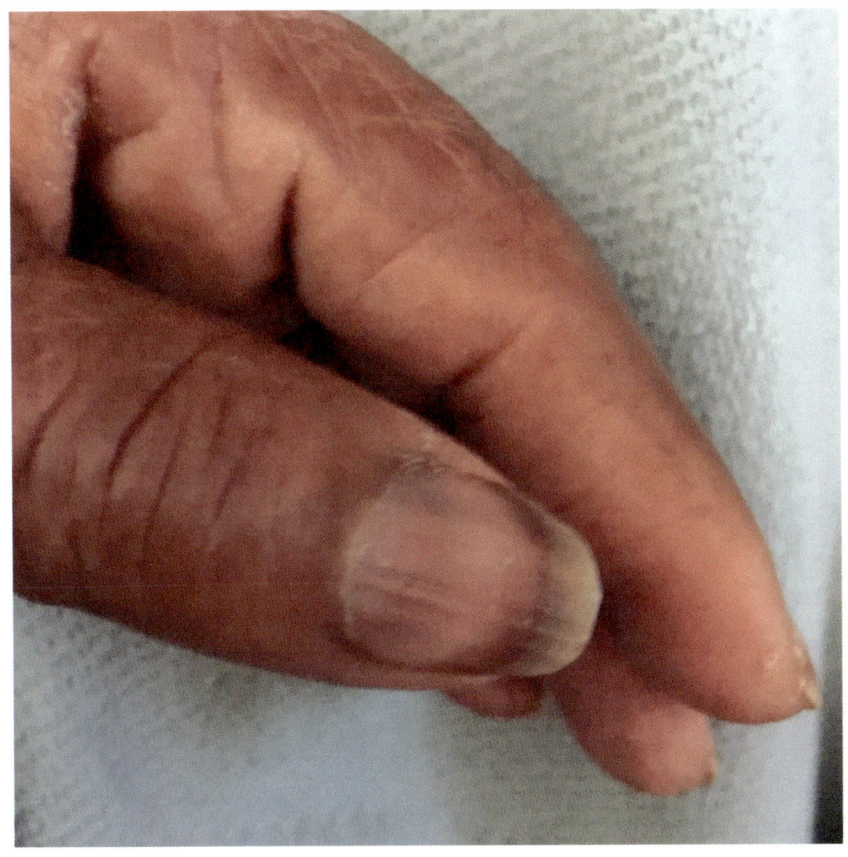

Case 17

Case 17

A 50 year-old woman presents to your office for a consultation. She has no known exposure to Human immunodeficiency virus infection or its treatment. What is the most likely cause of her nail findings?

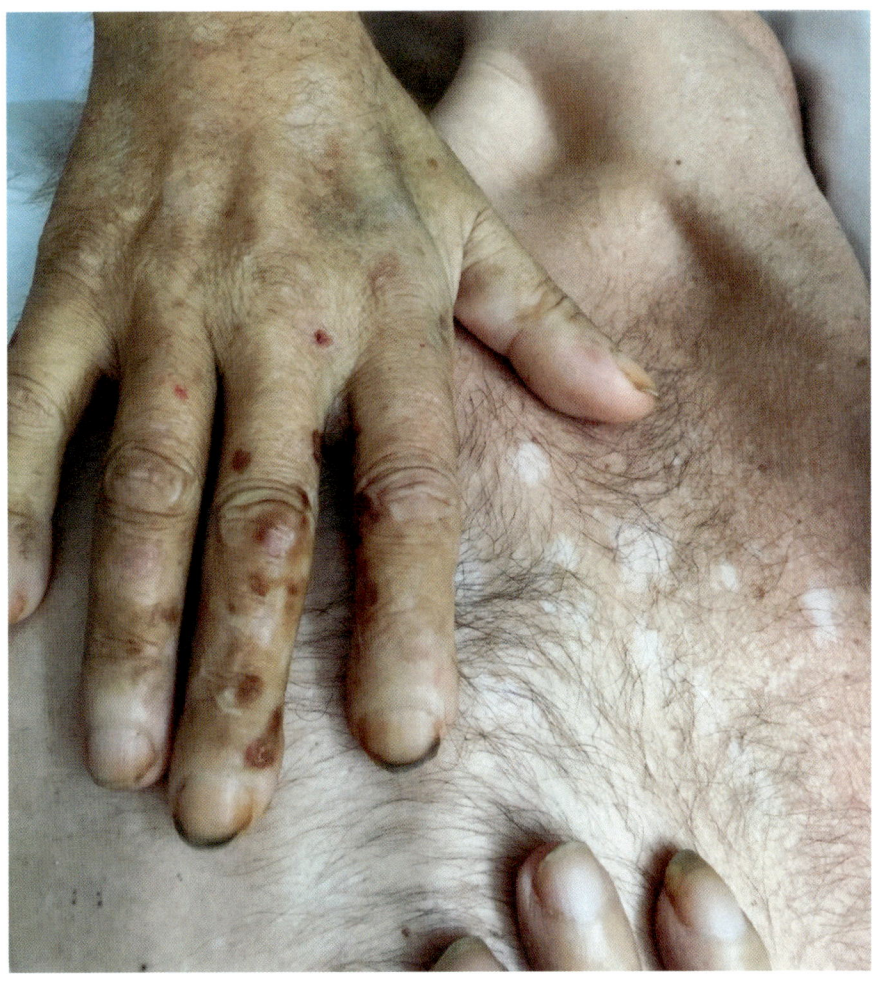

Case 18

Case 18

A 44 year-old man is brought to the ED in a coma. How do you explain the skin findings on his fingers and trunk? What is the likely cause of his unresponsive state?

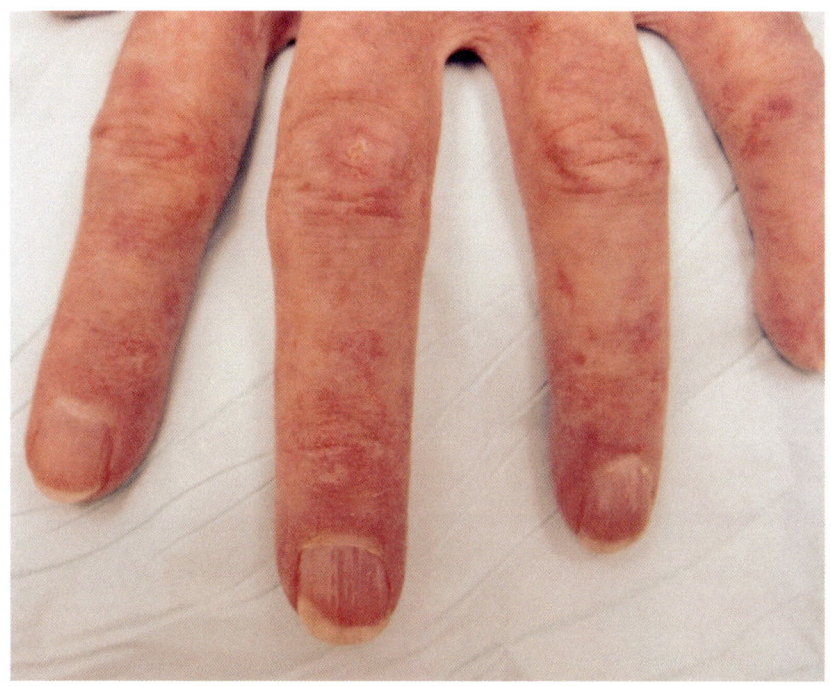

Case 19

Case 19

A 72 year-old woman presents to your office with symptoms of food getting stuck in her mid chest, cough, fatigue and weakness. She has to swallow liquids to help get the food down. She has noted an increase in the red dots over her fingers. What is the most likely explanation of her symptoms?

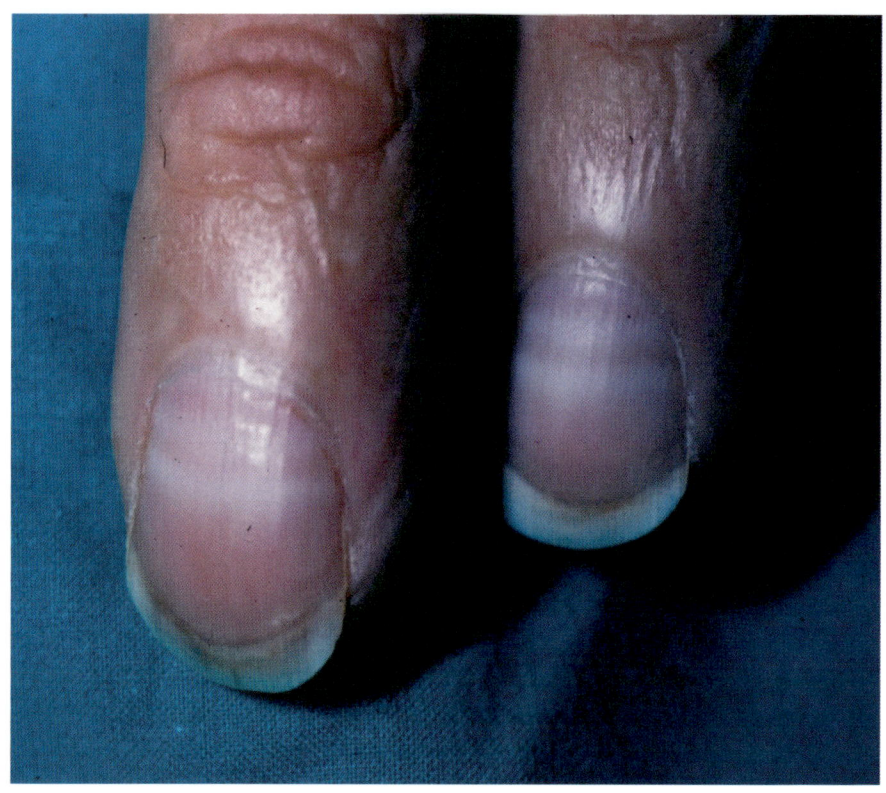

Case 20

Case 20

What is the cause of these nails change in this 60-year-old man?

How long have they been present?

Chapter 10

Case Answers and Discussion

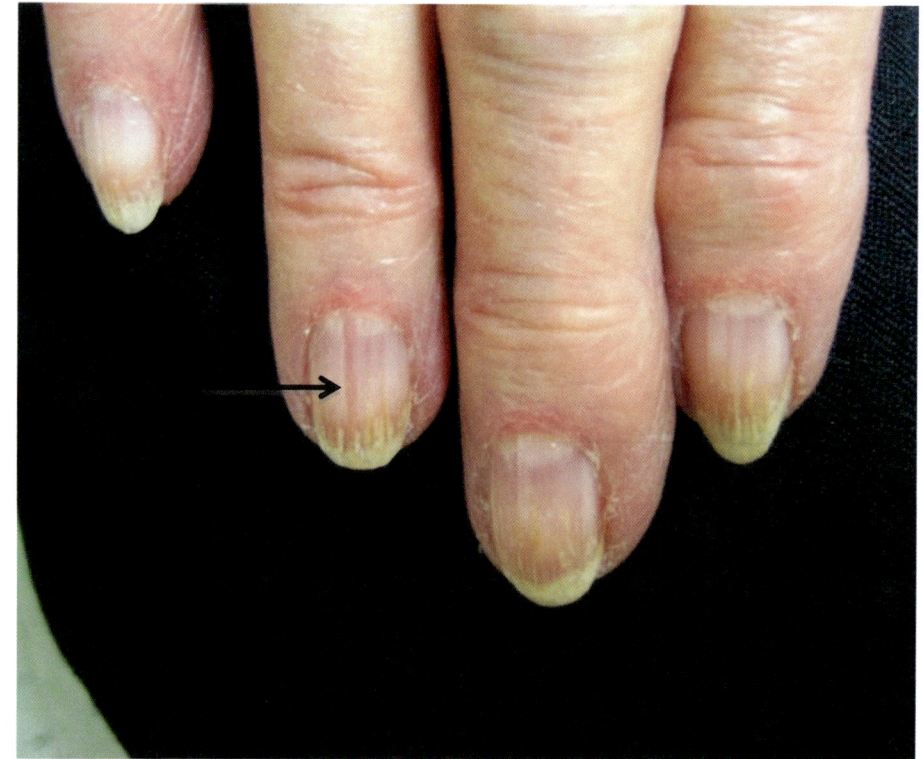

Case 1 Diabetes Mellitus with Peripheral Arterial Disease

Case 1 Diabetes Mellitus with Peripheral Arterial Disease

The key nail findings are yellowing and longitudinal ridges. The ridging suggests an endocrine problem while the yellowing can signify diabetes mellitus. <u>When you see yellow nails think of diabetes mellitus</u>. The redness around the cuticle is another clue. The longitudinal pink line on the ring finger (arrow) suggests peripheral arterial disease.

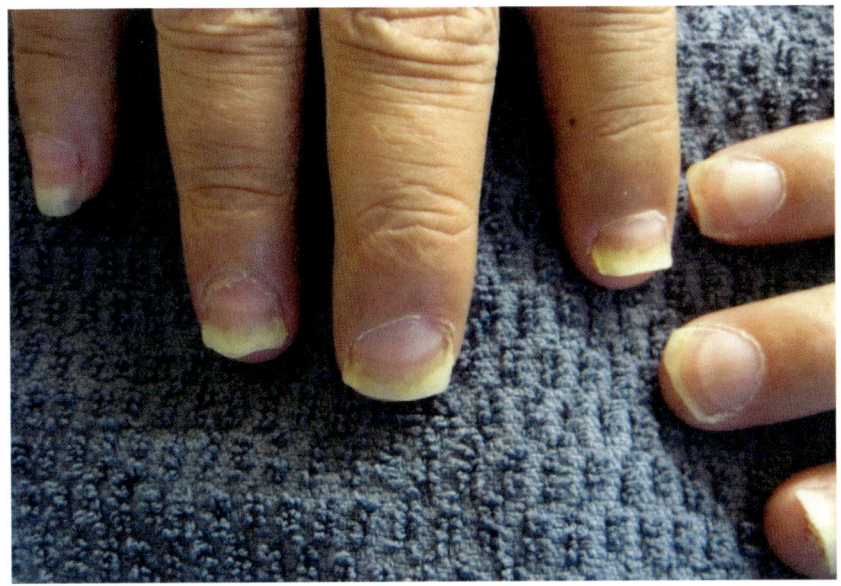

Case 2 Terry's half-and-half nails due to liver disease

Case 2 Liver disease with Terry's Half-and-Half nails

An initial observation is that the lunula appears large, but since no condition makes the lunula larger these must be Terry's half- and-half nails. They generally signify either chronic liver disease or chronic kidney disease. There is no convincing distal brown line below the free edge of the nail (which would imply chronic kidney disease) so these nails are likely the result of chronic liver disease with volume overload to explain the edema and possible ascites. There is also mild spooning suggesting nutrient deficiency.

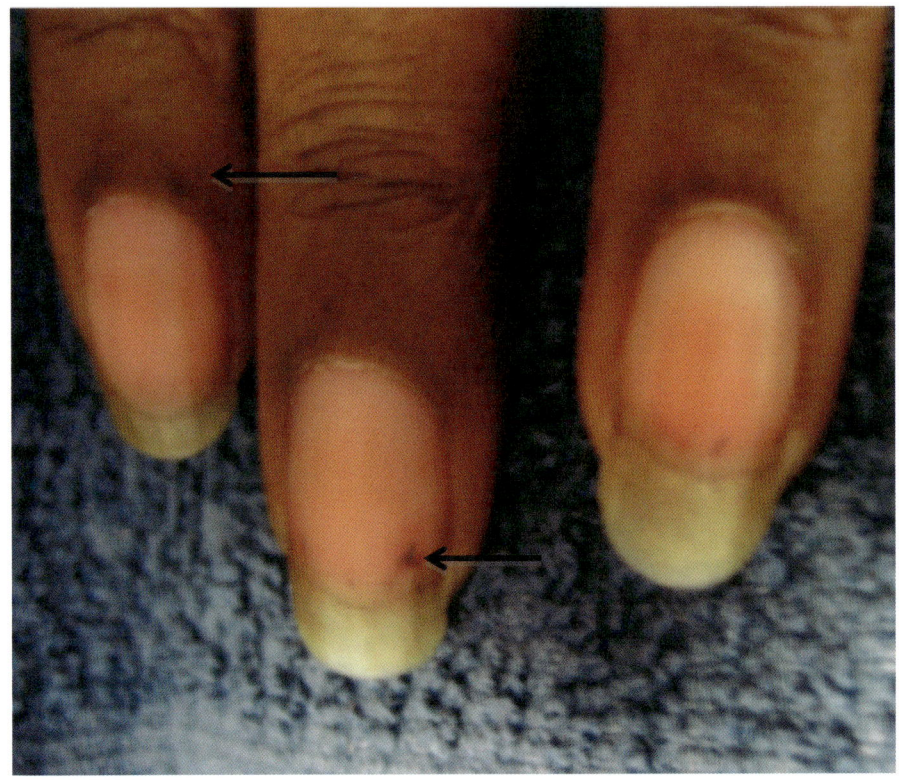

Case 3 Systemic Lupus Erythematosis with Splinter Hemorrhages

Case 3

Systemic Lupus Erythematosis with Splinter Hemorrhages

There are fat splinter hemorrhages and a periungal telangiectasia on the ring finger suggesting a connective tissue disease. A useful rule of thumb is to always consider SLE when bacterial endocarditis is in the differential diagnosis and vice versa. The lunula is absent implying anemia or malnutrition.

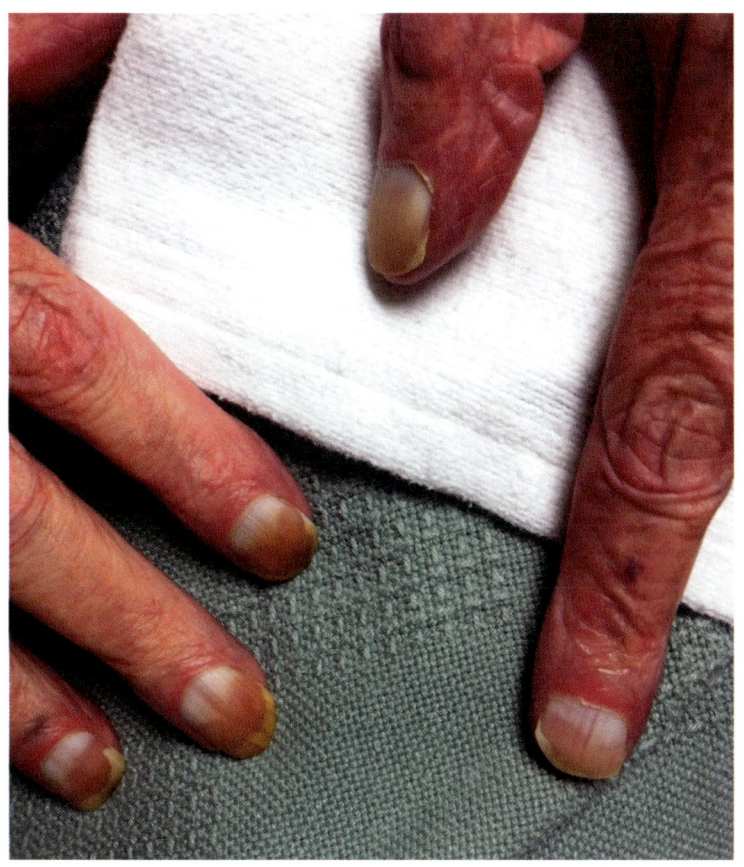

Case 4 Chronic kidney disease with secondary hyperthyroidism (Terry's half-and-half nails)

Case 4

Chronic Kidney disease with secondary hyperparathyroidism

These are Terry's half-and-half nails with the proximal portion of the nail being pale and the distal end pink. The dark brown line below the free edge of the nail suggests chronic kidney disease as the cause (See arrow). The nails have a subtle downward curvature that implies resorption of the distal phalange from hyperparathyroidism. There is also a brown, nicotine stain to the patient's right fingertips from cigarette smoking and longitudinal pink lines suggesting peripheral vascular disease.

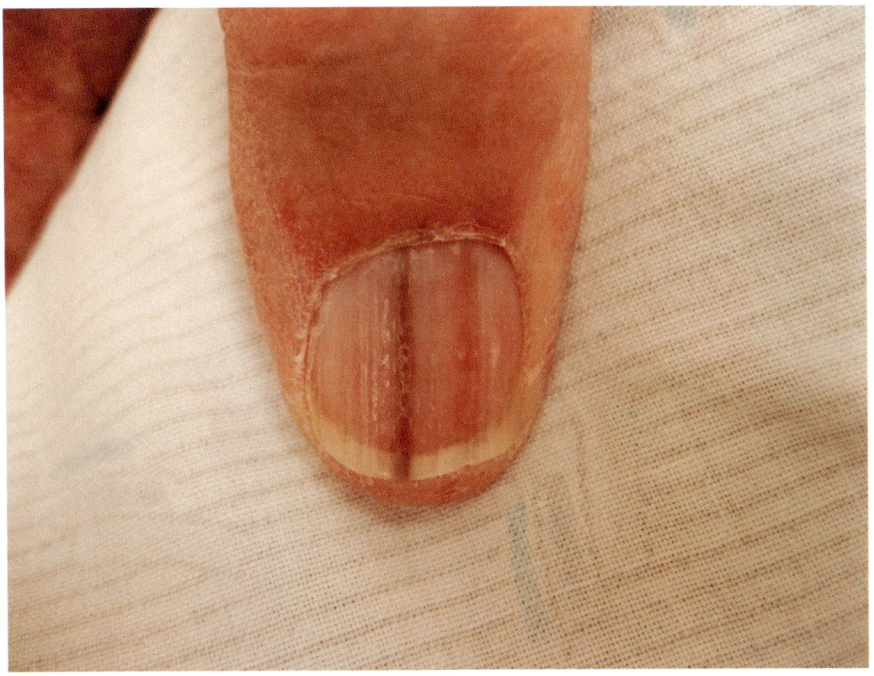

Case 5 Addison's disease

Case 5 Addison's Disease

The important observations are the longitudinal dark brown line implying a hyperpigmenting condition or trauma and the longitudinal ridges (beading) that suggests endocrine disorders. These findings along with his symptoms raise the possibility of adrenal insufficiency. Individuals with Addison's disease may have an increased sense of smell. There is also a longitudinal red line reflecting possible peripheral arterial disease. There is no cuticular nevus or mass to suggest melanoma.

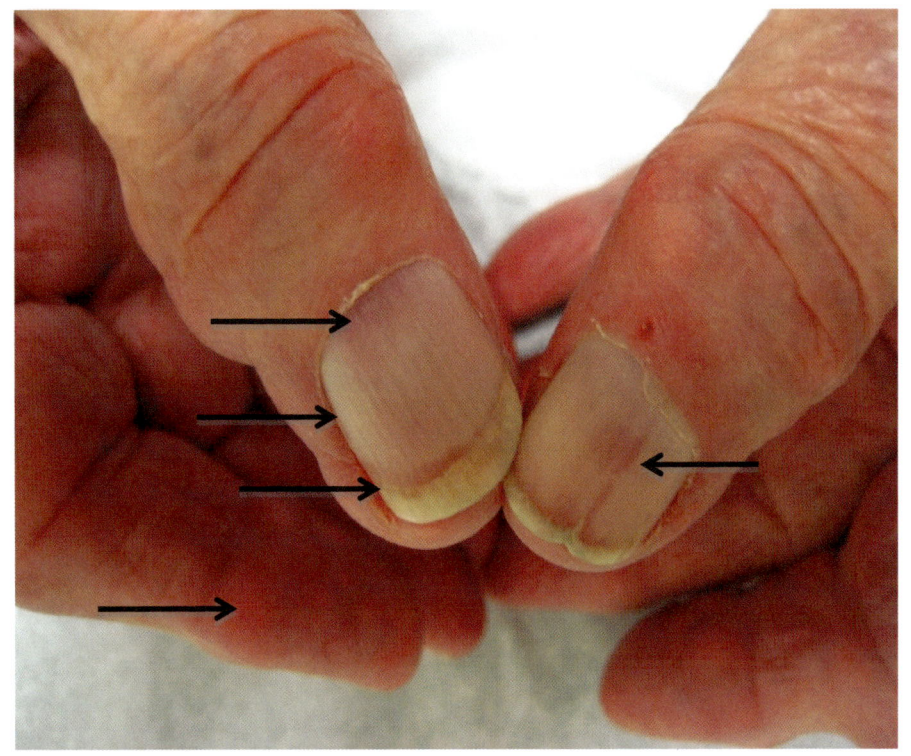

Case 6 Multiple Conditions shown on the nails

Case 6 Multiple conditions shown on the nails

1. Cardiac disease from the red lunula

2. Anemia from the overall pallor

3. Peripheral arterial disease reflected in the longitudinal red line

4. Chronic kidney disease from the distal transverse brown pigmentation

5. Gout from the subtle tophi on the fingertips and ankle discomfort

The red area below the cuticle on the left thumb is a scratch and is not a dilated capillary loop.

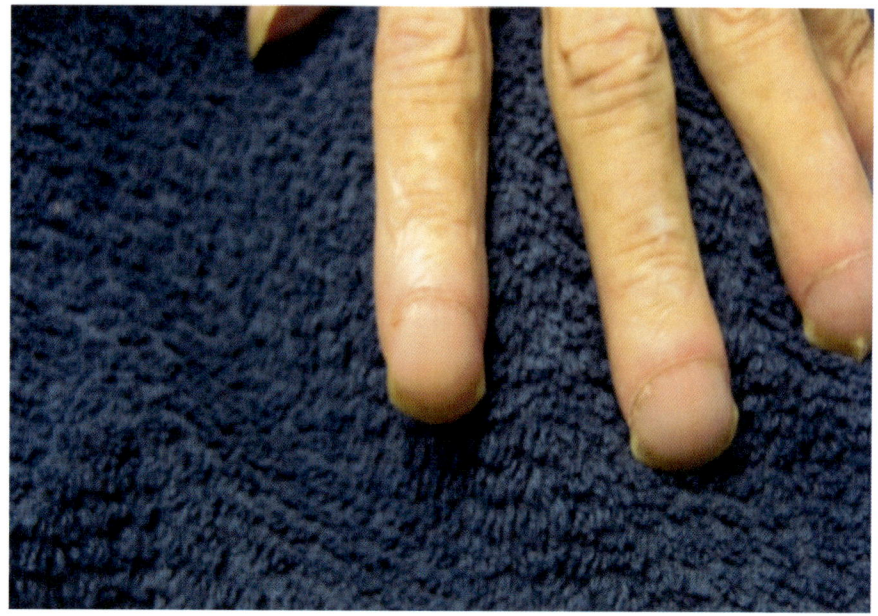

Case 7 Squamous cell cancer of the Esophagus

Case 7

Squamous cell cancer of the Esophagus

The extreme beaking of the nails implies resorption of the distal digit: In this particular case due to a parathyroid hormone-like substance produced by his malignancy. Many squamous cell cancers can produce PTHrP. The loss of the lunula confirms malnutrition or anemia. His symptom of dysphagia suggests the esophagus as a likely location of the malignancy although squamous cell cancer of any organ can produce PTHrP. Systemic sclerosis (scleroderma) is another consideration but seeing fine transverse wrinkles near the DIP joint makes this condition less likely. Often with systemic sclerosis the fingers look like they have dipped in paraffin.

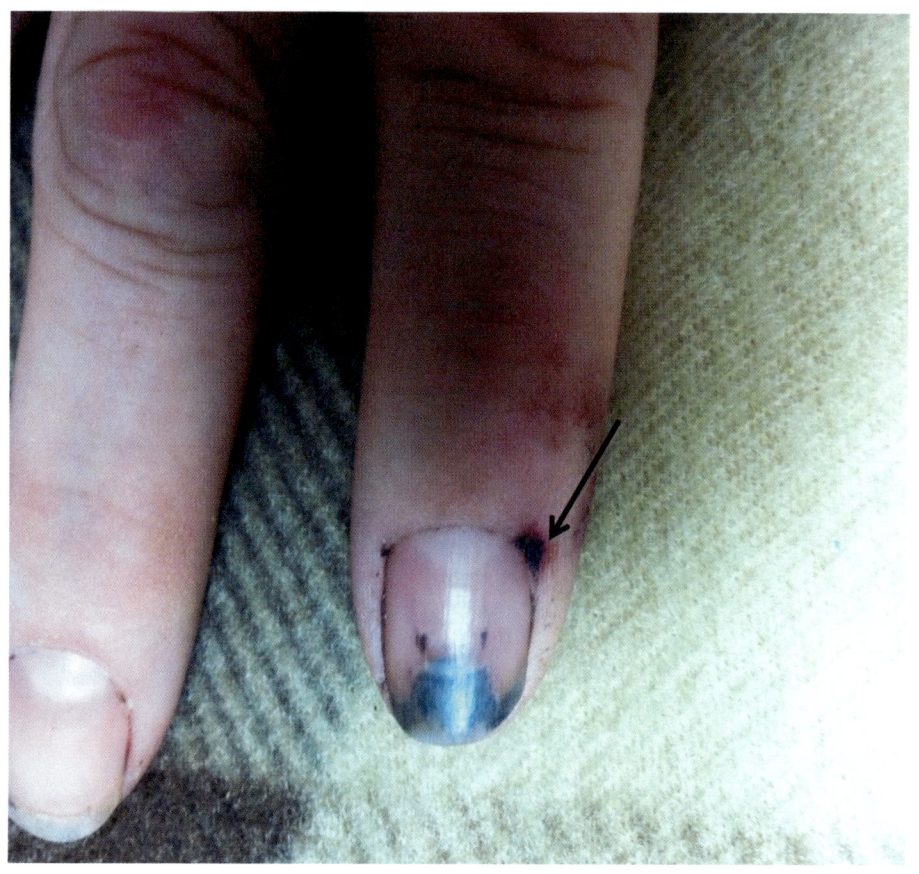

Case 8 Subacute Bacterial Endocarditis

Case 8 Sub Acute Bacterial Endocarditis

The periungal telangiectasias (See arrow) suggest one of four diagnoses: SLE, scleroderma, dermatomyositis, or systemic vasculitis. The skin over the fingers is not taut and hide-bound lowering the probability of scleroderma. The nail is destroyed so systemic vasculitis from SBE or systemic lupus is most likely. The classical teaching is that the rash of SLE tends to involve the skin between the knuckles and tends to spare the knuckles while dermatomyositis involves the skin over the knuckles and tend to spare the skin between the knuckles. Blood cultures grew gram-positive organisms.

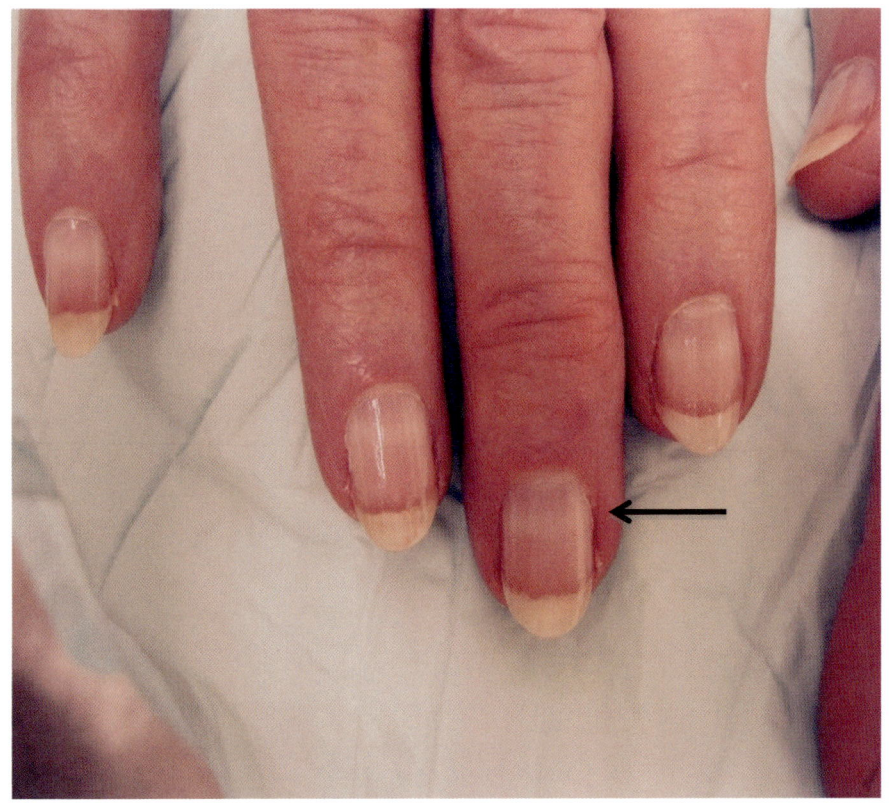

Case 9 Mee's line

Case 9 Mee's line of Acute Illness

There is a faint transverse white line about one third of the way up the nail implying an acute illness about two months ago. There is longitudinal ridging raising the possibility of an endocrine disorder and a distal brown line below the free edge of the nail suggesting possible chronic kidney disease. The nails have a glossy appearance of a recent manicure since the polish goes all the way to the cuticle. A recent manicure implies a sense of well-being. The lunula is faintly visible so anemia and malnutrition is less likely.

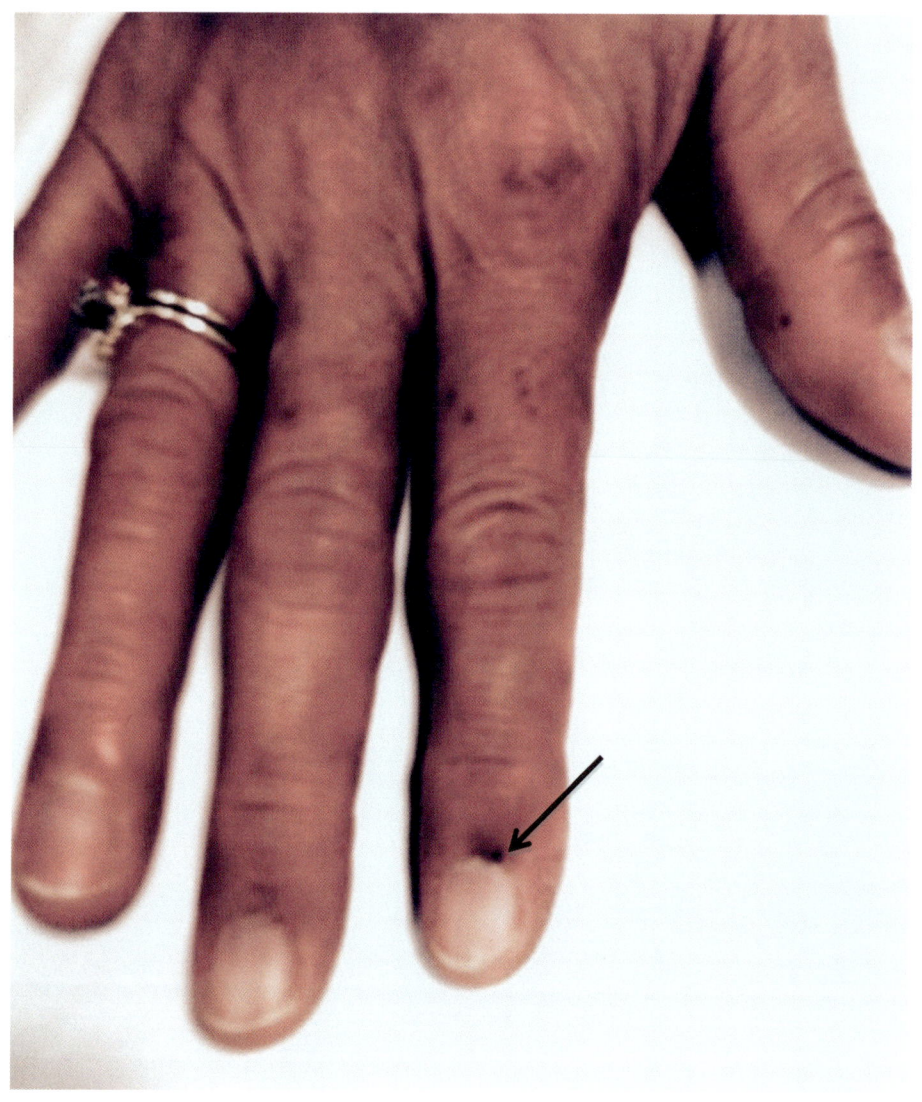

Case 10 Systemic Lupus Erythematosis

Case 10 Systemic Lupus Erythematosis

The significant atrophy of the cuticle and the periungal telangiectasias (See arrow) suggest autoimmune disease. There are fine transverse wrinkles making scleraderma less likely. The rash is tending to spare the knuckles, which increases the likelihood of SLE over dermatomyositis (a useful rule of thumb).

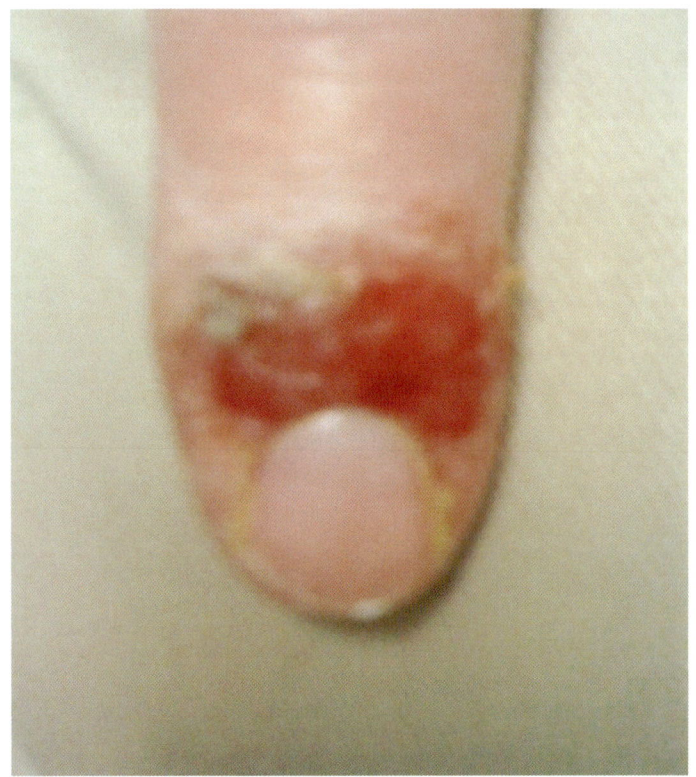

Case 11 Acute Paronychia

Case 11 Acute Paronychia

The redness with crusting and swelling is characteristic of acute paronychia. Acute paronychia is usually caused by a bacterial infection. Water exposure, foreign body, aggressive manicure or pulling a hangnail each predispose to paronychial infection. Six weeks is considered the cut off between acute and chronic paronychias.

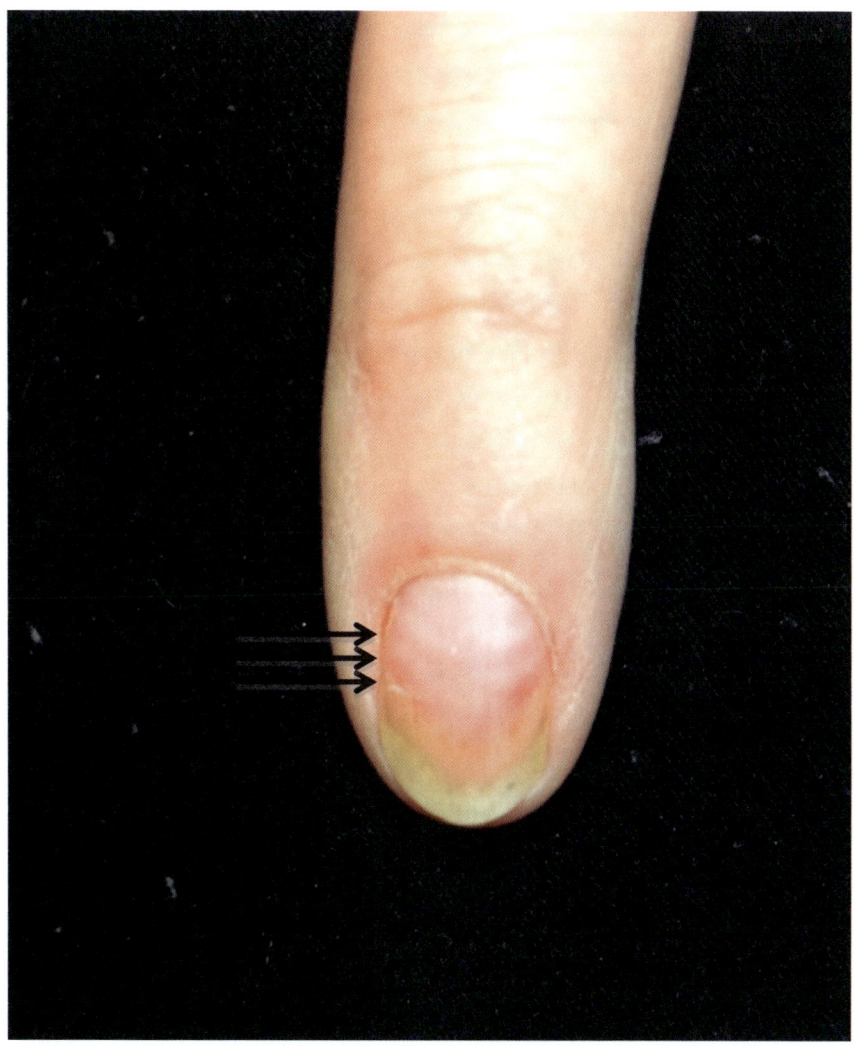

Case 12 Cyclic Chemotherapy (multiple Mee's lines)

Case 12 Cyclical Chemotherapy

The lunula is indistinct and there are at least three transverse white lines evenly spaced along the nail roughly at one-month intervals. While separate, significant illnesses could explain the finding, the most likely inference is cyclical chemotherapy for malignancy. These are sometimes called a "ladder" of Mee's lines.

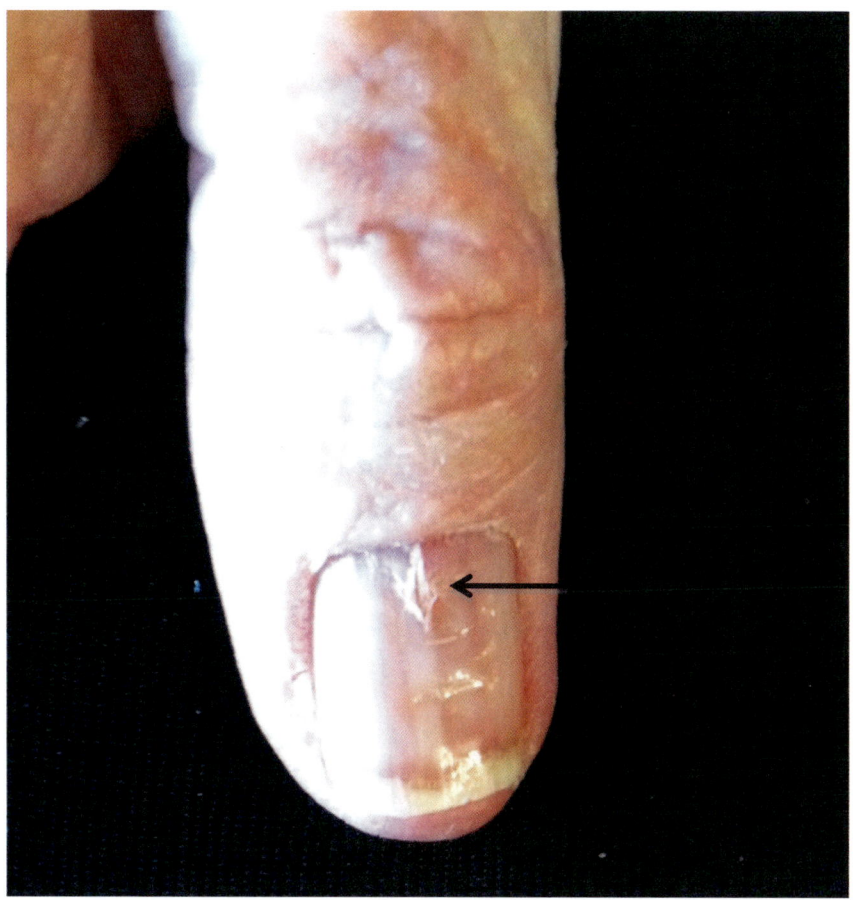

Case 13 Subungal Fibroma

Case 13 Subungal Fibroma

The nail is distorted but the cuticle is intact. The faint transverse lines above the mass suggest trauma to the cuticle. The most likely condition is a benign subungal fibroma.

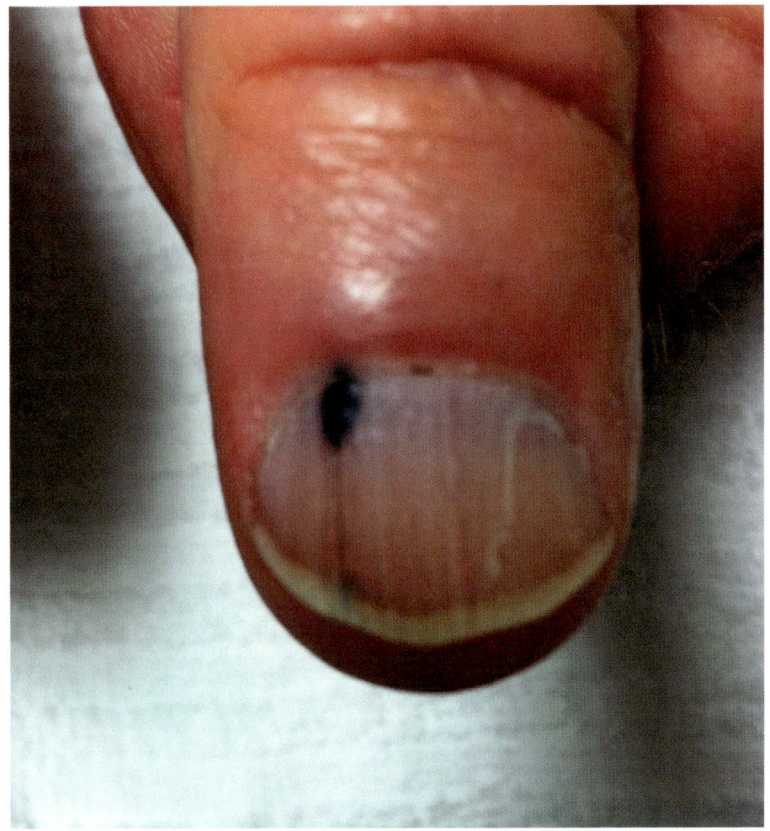

Case 14 Subungal Melanoma

Case 14 Malignant Melanoma

The key finding is the obvious black discoloration of the proximal thumbnail with a faint hyperpigmented longitudinal brown line. The cuticle is involved. Any lesion of this nature should be immediately biopsied. The differential diagnosis would also include a large splinter hemorrhage.

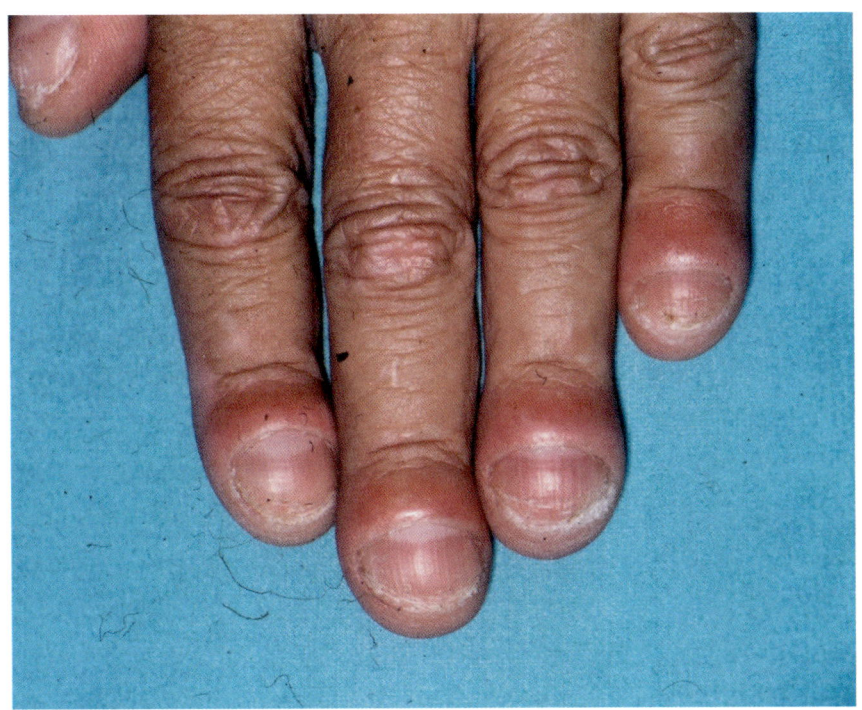

Case 15 Clubbing from Lung Cancer

Case 15 Clubbing from Lung Cancer

The distal caliber of the fingers is larger than the proximal caliber so these fingers show clubbing. About 80% of clubbing is due to a pulmonary or cardiac cause. The patient's significant weight loss suggests occult malignancy and the cough points to a lung site rather than the GI tract. The ragged tips of these nails would also raise the consideration of thyrotoxicosis (which can also cause clubbing) but in this case a lung cancer was discovered.

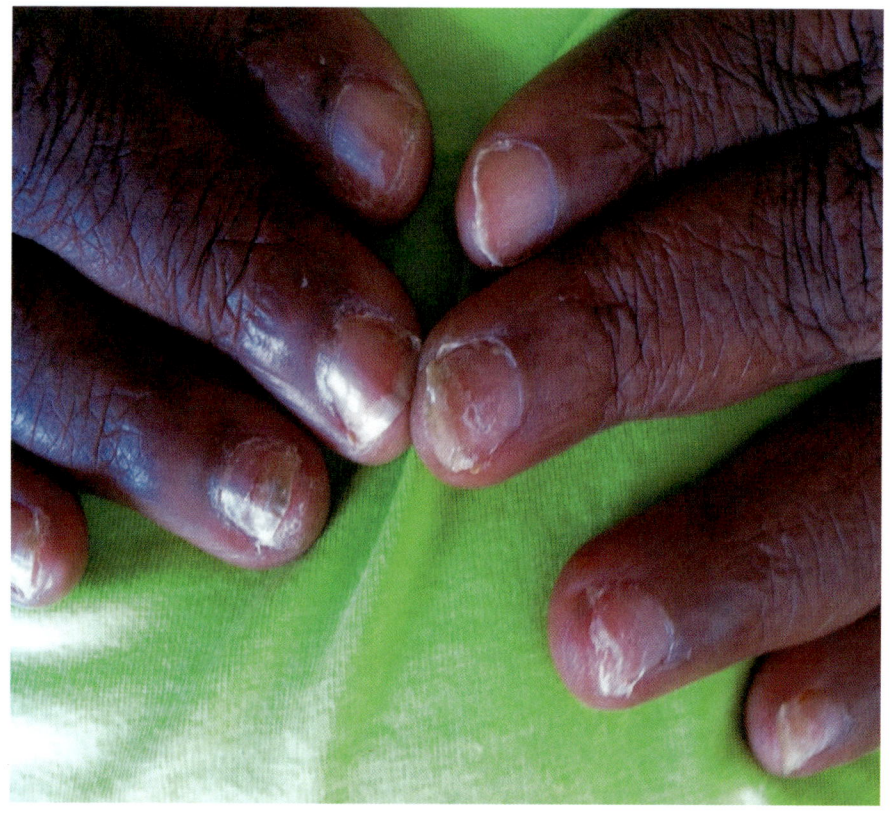

Case 16 Voriconazole Nails

Case 16 Vorconazole Nail Changes

The key findings in this image include the dull, rough nail surface with scaling of the body of the nail. Toxic exposures or autoimmune diseases are considerations. Voriconazole given for fungal disease in ill immunosuppressed patients can produce alopecia and these nail changes. When the medication is stopped the hair and nails can regrow.

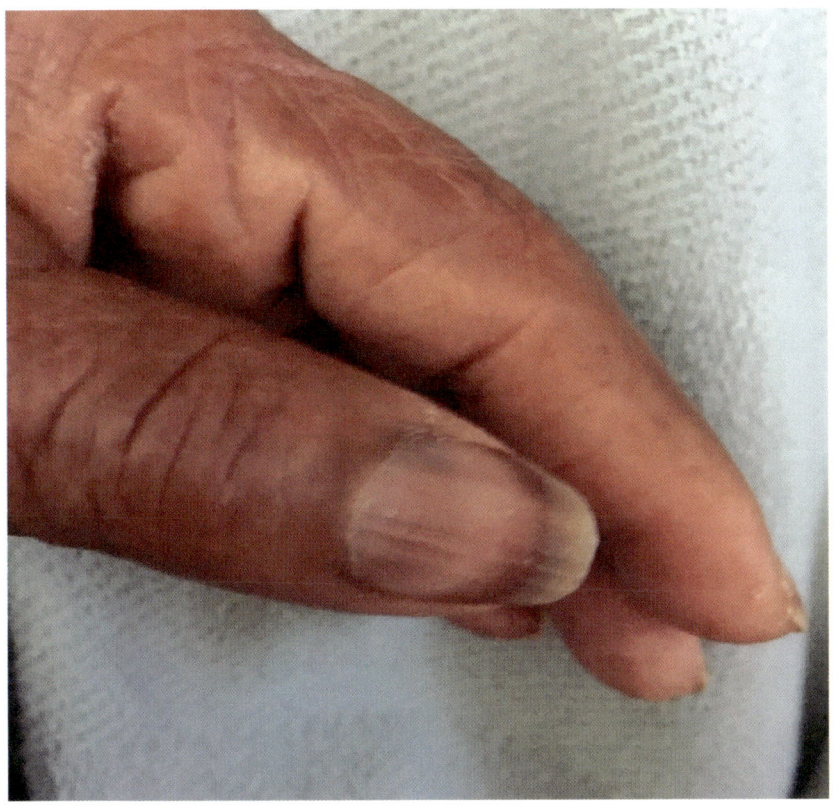

Case 17 Brown nails from hydroxyurea

Case 17 Brown Nails from Hydroxyurea

The nails show longitudinal ridges and broad transverse bands of hyperpigmentation suggesting cyclical exposure to a agent that produces brown discoloration called melanonychia. While endocrine disorders such as Addison disease, Cushing disease or hyperthyroidism are possible, these conditions usually produce longitudinal rather than transverse pigmentation. In this case the patient had received hydroxyurea treatments over two month intervals.

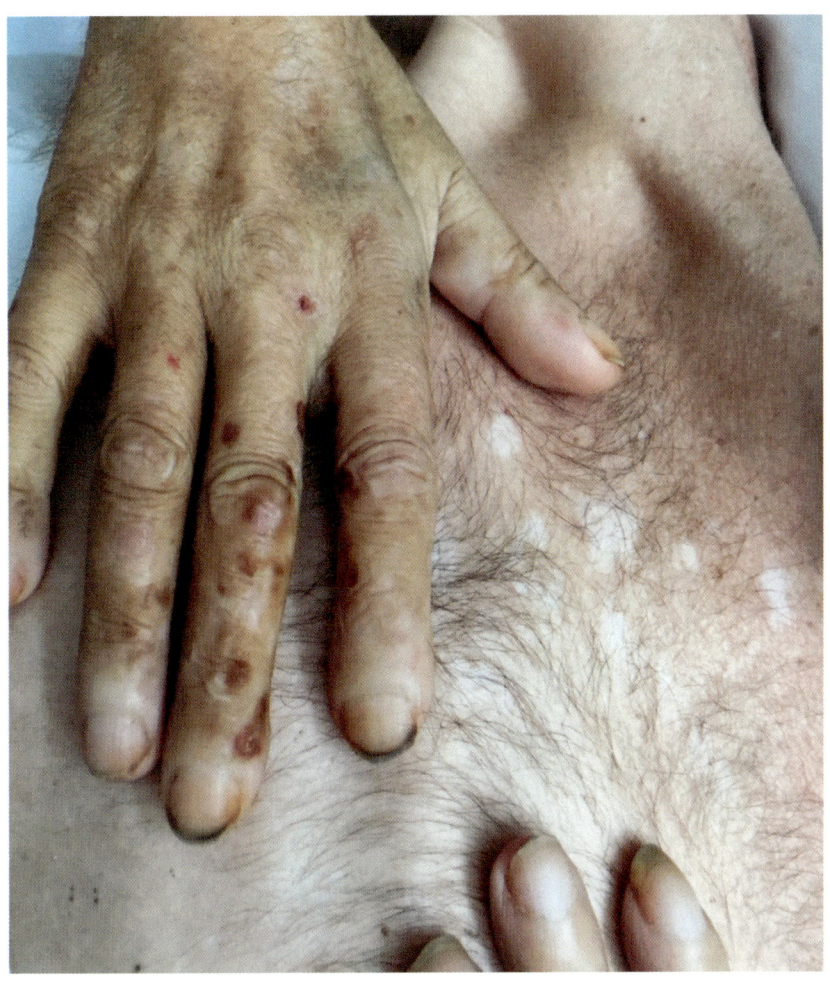

Case 18 Cigarette burns from chronic narcotic use

Case 18 Cigarette burns from chronic narcotic use

There are fresh cigarette burns on the fingers and old burns on the trunk. These are produced when a narcotic user nods off while smoking and is oblivious to the burn. These are signs of significant muscle wasting and the nails are dull and pale with a loss of the lunula implying anemia and malnutrition. His unresponsive state in this case was due to narcotic overdose.

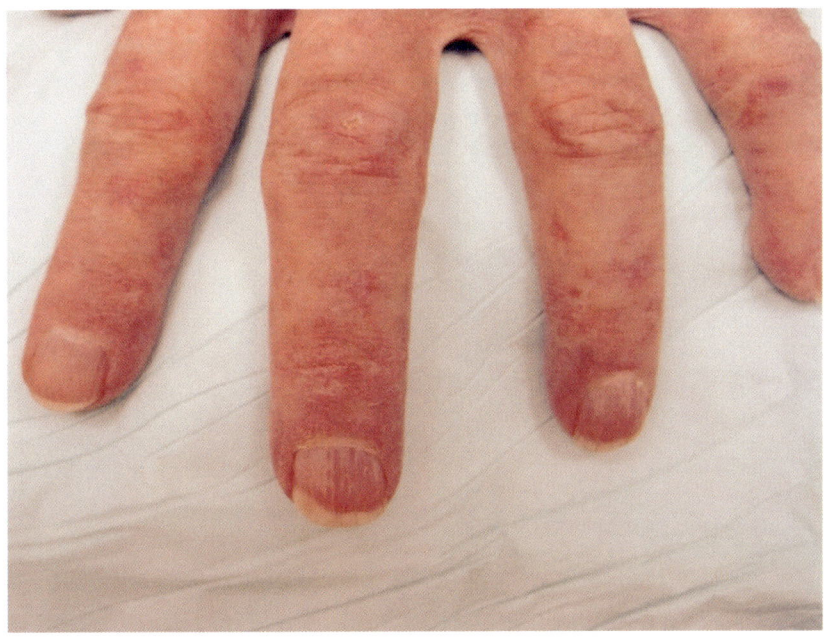

Case 19 CREST syndrome

Case 19 CREST syndrome

The name CREST refers to the findings of calcinosis, Raynaud's phenomenon, esophageal dysmotility, sclerodactyly, and telangiectasia. It is a form of connective tissue disease related to systemic sclerosis. The nails show atrophy of the cuticle with periungal telangiectasia. There are telangiectasias over the fingers and loss of the transverse creases. Her swallowing symptoms are classical for esophageal dysmotility. Laboratory studies showed anti-centromere antibodies.

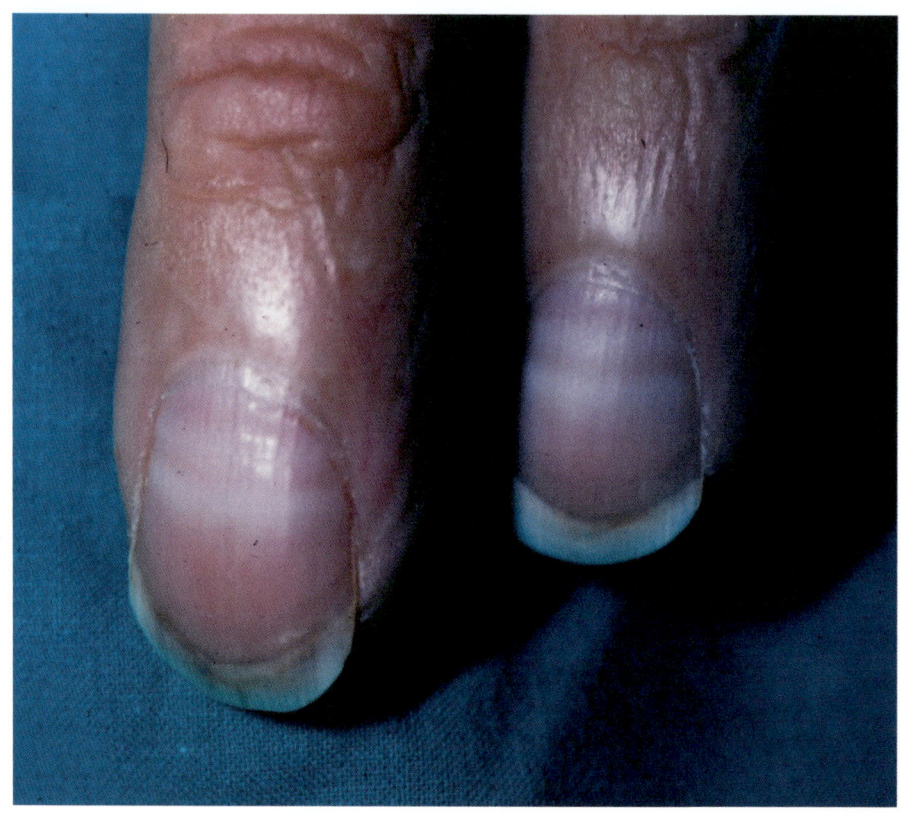

Case 20 Muehrcke's lines of hypoalbuminemia

Case 20 Severe Malnutrition

The nails show irregular parallel transverse lines called Muehrcke's lines, which are caused by very low serum albumin. Edema under the nail produces Muehrcke's lines and they disappear when the albumin rises. Because the lines are not in the nail itself they do not migrate up the nail over time. As a result, the chronicity of the malnutrition cannot be estimated with precision. Loss of the lunula also reflects a low serum albumin, possible anemia and malnutrition.

Fingernail Bibliography

NAIL POLISH

Cruz MJ; Baudrier T; Cunha AP; Ferreira O; Azevedo F. Severe onychodystrophy caused by allergic contact dermatitis to acrylates in artificial nails. Cutaneous & Ocular Toxicology. 30(4):323-4, 2011 Dec.

Mendelsohn E; Hagopian A; Hoffman K; Butt CM; Lorenzo A; Congleton J; Webster TF; Stapleton HM. Nail polish as a source of exposure to triphenyl phosphate. Environment International. 86:45-51, 2016 Jan.

Hinkelbein J; Koehler H; Genzwuerker HV; Fiedler F.Artificial acrylic finger nails may alter pulse oximetry measurement. Resuscitation. 74(1):75-82, 2007 Jul.

Rodden AM; Spicer L; Diaz VA; Steyer TE. Does fingernail polish affect pulse oximeter readings?. Comment in: Intensive Crit Care Nurs. 2008 Feb;24(1):4-5; PMID: 17689251 Intensive & Critical Care Nursing. 23(1):51-5, 2007 Feb.

Hakverdioglu Yont G; Akin Korhan E; Dizer B.The effect of nail polish on pulse oximetry readings. Intensive & Critical Care Nursing. 30(2):111-5, 2014 Apr.

LUNULA

Sandre MK; Rohekar S; Guenther L.GRS Nubes Supra Lunam, a New Lunula Shape. Journal of Cutaneous Medicine & Surgery. 19(6):528-9, 2015 Nov-Dec.

Zhou H; Zhao Y; Yu X; Chen S; Chen D; Wang W; Wang Z; Wu X; Zhang Z.The association between absent lunula and depression in depressive outpatients: a case-control study. Psychiatry Research. 205(1-2):176-8, 2013 Jan 30. Our study found that depression was associated with absent lunula, and severe depression was associated with a greater number of absent lunula.

Tosti A, Paoluzzi P, Baran R Doubled nail of the thumb: a rare form of polydactyly, Dermatology 184: 216–218, 1992.

NAIL SHAPE

NAIL CLUBBING

Fischer DS, Singer DH, Feldman SM Clubbing, a review, with emphasis on hereditary acropachy, *Medicine* **43**:459–479, 1964.

Pallares-Sanmartin A; Leiro-Fernandez V; Cebreiro TL; Botana-Rial M; Fernandez-Villar A.Validity and reliability of the Schamroth sign for the diagnosis of clubbing. JAMA. 304(2):159-61, 2010 Jul 14.

Dickinson CJ, Martin JF Megakaryocytes and platelet clumps as the cause of finger clubbing, *Lancet* **ii:**1434–1435, 1987

Nakamura J; Halliday NA; Fukuba E; Radjenovic A; Tanner SF; Emery P; McGonagle D; Tan AL. The microanatomic basis of finger clubbing - a high-resolution magnetic resonance imaging study. Journal of Rheumatology. 41(3):523-7, 2014 Mar.

BEAU'S LINES

Ryu H; Lee HJ.Beau's lines of the fingernails. American Journal of the Medical Sciences. 349(4):363, 2015 Apr.

Park, Juhee; Li, Kapsok.Multiple Beau's lines.New England Journal of Medicine. 362(20):e63, 2010 May 20.

Lee, Yong-Ju; Yun, Seok-Kweon. Unilateral Beau's lines associatd with a fingertip crushing injury. Journal of Dermatology. 32(11):914-6, 2005 Nov.

Miyoshi I; Kubota T; Taguchi H.Beau's lines after chemotherapy for ALL.Internal Medicine. 46(1):61, 2007.

MECHANICAL STRESSORS

Olszewska M; Wu JZ; Slowinska M; Rudnicka L.The 'PDA nail': traumatic nail dystrophy in habitual users of personal digital assistants. American Journal of Clinical Dermatology. 10(3):193-6, 2009.

Wu, Jashin J.Habit tic deformity secondary to guitar playing. Dermatology Online Journal. 15(3):16, 2009.

Latham L; Langley R. Dermacase. Can you identify this condition? Median canaliform nail dystrophy. Canadian Family Physician. 59(5):511, 513, 2013 May.

Sano H; Ichioka S .Influence of mechanical forces as a part of nail configuration. Dermatology. 225(3):210-4, 2012.

Sano H; Ogawa R. Role of mechanical forces in hand nail configuration asymmetry in hemiplegia: an analysis of four hundred thumb nails.Dermatology. 226(4):315-8, 2013.

Sano H; Shionoya K; Ogawa R.Effect of mechanical forces on finger nail curvature: an analysis of the effect of occupation on finger nails. Dermatologic Surgery. 40(4):441-5, 2014 Apr.

NAIL SURFACE

Lee YB; Cheon MS; Eun YS; Park HJ; Cho BK.Elkonyxis in association with washboard nail and 20-nail dystrophy. International Journal of Dermatology. 53(1):e11-3, 2014 Jan.

NAILS AND GLAUCOMA

Pasquale LR; Hanyuda A; Ren A; Giovingo M; Greenstein SH; Cousins C; Patrianakos T; Tanna AP; Wanderling C; Norkett W; Wiggs JL; Green K; Kang JH; Knepper PA.

Nailfold Capillary Abnormalities in Primary Open-Angle Glaucoma: A Multisite Study. Investigative Ophthalmology & Visual Science. 56(12):7021-8, 2015 Nov.

NAIL COLORATION

André J, Lateur N. Pigmented nail disorders. Dermatol Clin 24:329-339, 2006

Baran R, Kechijian P Longitudinal melanonychia (melanonychia striata): diagnosis and management, J Am Acad Dermatol 21:1165–1175, 1989.

Daniel CR Nail pigmentation abnormalities, Dermatol Clin 3:431–443, 1985.

Kumar R; Zawar V. Longitudinal leukonychia in Hailey-Hailey Disease: a sign not to be missed. Dermatology Online Journal. 14(3):17, 2008.

A 54-year-old male presented with a painful, erythematous, fissured plaque involving the left groin and adjacent scrotal skin. In addition, he exhibited white longitudinal bands and ridges on his fingernails, more prominent on thumb nails. Skin biopsy from the left groin confirmed the diagnosis of chronic familial benign pemphigus (Hailey-Hailey disease). To the best of our knowledge, this is the first case report from India in which we have described nail involvement in Hailey-Hailey disease.

Saraya T; Ariga M; Kurai D; Takeshita N; Honda K; Goto H. Terry's nails as a part of aging. Internal Medicine. 47(6):567-8, 2008.

Ceyhan AM; Yildirim M; Bircan HA; Karayigit DZ.Transverse leukonychia (Mees' lines) associated with docetaxel.Journal of Dermatology. 37(2):188-9, 2010 Feb.

Stanifer J; Mehta R; Mettu N; Sanders J; Setji N.Muehrcke's lines as a diagnostic clue to increased catabolism and a severe systemic disease state. American Journal of the Medical Sciences. 342(4):331, 2011 Oct.

Kluger N; Naud M; Frances P.Toenails melanonychia induced by hydroxyurea. Presse Medicale. 41(4):444-5, 2012 Apr.

Luigetti M; Conte A; Bisogni G; Del Grande A; Sabatelli M.'White nails'. Skin changes in POEMS syndrome. European Neurology. 73(1-2):89, 112, 2015.

Baran B; Soyer OM; Karaca C.Terry's nail: an overlooked physical finding in cirrhosis. Comment in: Hepatobiliary Pancreat Dis Int. 2014 Jun;13(3):332; PMID: 24919619 Comment in: Hepatobiliary Pancreat Dis Int. 2014 Jun;13(3):332-3; PMID: 24919620 Hepatobiliary & Pancreatic Diseases Int. 12(1):109, 2013 Feb.

Poppe LM; Brocker EB; Trautmann A.The one-nail brown band: macro- and micro-morphology. Acta Dermato-Venereologica. 93(4):479-80, 2013 Jul 6

Chadha S; Nannapaneni S; Shetty V; Shani J.Half-and-half nail.American Journal of the Medical Sciences. 346(6):513, 2013 Dec.

Nia AM; Ederer S; Dahlem KM; Gassanov N; Er F.Terry's nails: a window to systemic diseases.American Journal of Medicine. 124(7):602-4, 2011 Jul.

Pellegrino, M; Taddeucci, P; Mei, S; Peccianti, C; Fimiani, M.Half-and-half nail in a patient with Crohn's disease. Journal of the European Academy of Dermatology & Venereology. 24(11):1366-7, 2010 Nov.

Morrison-Bryant, Maya; Gradon, Jeremy D.Muehrcke's lines. New England Journal of Medicine. 357(9):917, 2007 Aug 30.

Dalle S; Ronger-Savle S; Cicale L; Balme B; Thomas L.A blue-gray subungual discoloration.Archives of Dermatology. 143(7):937-42, 2007 Jul.

Verma P; Mahajan G. Verma, P; Mahajan, G.Idiopathic 'Half and half' nails.Journal of the European Academy of Dermatology & Venereology. 29(7):1452, 2015 Jul.

Herbers AH; Gerlag PG. Herbers, A H E; Gerlag, P G G. Bluish-grey pigmentation of fingernails, gingiva, teeth and peri-oral region. Minocycline. Netherlands Journal of Medicine. 62(2):58, 65, 2004 Feb.

Huan, T C; Ho, C L. Blue-black discoloration of the nails associated with gefitinib. Acta Clinica Belgica. 66(1):72, 2011 Jan-Feb.

Leung AK; McLeod DR .Familial melanonychia striata.Journal of the National Medical Association. 100(6):743-5, 2008 Jun.

Yang CS; Robinson-Bostom L.Images in clinical medicine. Lindsay's nails in chronic kidney disease.New England Journal of Medicine. 372(18):1748, 2015 Apr 30

Chiriac A; Brzezinski P; Foia L; Marincu I.Chloronychia: green nail syndrome caused by Pseudomonas aeruginosa in elderly persons. Clinical Interventions In Aging. 10:265-7, 2015.

Grazzini M; Rossari S; Gori A; Corciova S; Guerriero G; Lotti T; De Giorgi V..Subungueal pigmented lesions: warning for dermoscopic melanoma diagnosis. European Journal of Dermatology. 21(2):286-7, 2011 Mar-Apr.

Teive HA; Munhoz RP.Rotigotine-induced nail dyschromia in a patient with Parkinson disease.Neurology. 76(18):1605, 2011 May 3.

Huan TC; Ho CL. Blue-black discoloration of the nails associated with gefitinib. Acta Clinica Belgica. 66(1):72, 2011 Jan-Feb.

ONYCHOLYSIS

Baran R, Badillet G Primary onycholysis of the big toenails. A review of 113 cases, *Br J Dermatol* 106:526–534, 1982.

Kechijian P Onycholysis of the fingernails: evaluation and management, J Am Acad Dermatol 12:552–560, 1985

Levine, Norman.Levine,Norman. University of Arizona Health Sciences Center, Tucson, AZ, USA. Separation of nail plate from nail bed. There is no previous history of other skin conditions. Geriatrics. 61(2):17, 2006 Feb.

Umanoff N; Werner B; Rady PL; Tyring S; Carlson JA.Persistent toenail onycholysis associated with Beta-papillomavirus infection of the nail bed. American Journal of Dermatopathology. 37(4):329-33, 2015 Apr.

Lau CP; Hui P; Chan TC.Docetaxel-induced nail toxicity: a case of severe onycholysis and topic review. [Review] Chinese Medical Journal. 124(16):2559-60, 2011 Aug..

NAIL BEDS

Fehrenbacher V; Blackburn E. Fehrenbacher, Victor; Blackburn, Ethan.Nail bed injury. [Review]Journal of Hand Surgery - American Volume. 40(3):581-2, 2015 Mar.

Hatami M; Naftolin F; Khatamee MA.Abnormal fingernail beds following carbon monoxide poisoning: a case report and review of the literature. [Review] Journal of Medical Case Reports [Electronic Resource]. 8:263, 2014.

The fingernail tips were altered and appeared as if a bite had been taken out of their distal borders. The changes in the tips of her fingernails were significant, but they completely disappeared eight weeks later without any additional treatment.

Yamamoto S; Harada K; Ando N; Kawamura T; Shibagaki N; Tanaka M; Shimada S.Nodular melanoma on the hyponychium: clinical and dermoscopic features. Journal of Dermatology. 41(3):277-8, 2014 Mar.

PSORIASIS

Sandre MK; Rohekar S; Guenther L.Psoriatic Nail Changes Are Associated With Clinical Outcomes in Psoriatic Arthritis. Journal of Cutaneous Medicine & Surgery. 19(4):367-76, 2015 Jul-Aug.

Sandre MK; Rohekar S.Psoriatic arthritis and nail changes: exploring the relationship. [Review] Seminars in Arthritis & Rheumatism. 44(2):162-9, 2014 Oct.

Brazzelli V; Carugno A; Alborghetti A; Grasso V; Cananzi R; Fornara L; De Silvestri A; Borroni G. Prevalence, severity and clinical features of psoriasis in fingernails and toenails in adult patients: Italian experience. Journal of the European Academy of Dermatology & Venereology. 26(11):1354-9, 2012 Nov.

CONNECTIVE TISSUE DISEASE

Tunc SE; Ertam I; Pirildar T; Turk T; Ozturk M; Doganavsargil E.Nail changes in connective tissue diseases: do nail changes provide clues for the diagnosis?. Journal of the European Academy of Dermatology & Venereology. 21(4):497-503, 2007 Apr.

SYSTEMIC SCLEROSIS

Mizutani H, Mizutani T, Okada H *et al* Round fingerpad sign: an early sign of scleroderma, *J Am Acad Dermatol* 24: 67–69, 1991.

Wildt, M; Hesselstrand, R; Akesson, A; Scheja, A.Simple counting of nailfold capillary density in suspected systemic sclerosis - 9 years' experience.Scandinavian Journal of Rheumatology. 36(6):452-7, 2007 Nov-Dec.

Hofstee, H M A; Vonk Noordegraaf, A; Voskuyl, A E; Dijkmans, B A C; Postmus, P E; Smulders, Y M; Serne, E H.Nailfold capillary density is associated with the presence and severity of pulmonary arterial hypertension in systemic sclerosis.Annals of the

Rheumatic Diseases. 68(2):191-5, 2009 Feb.

Batticciotto A; Atzeni F; Foglia S; Antivalle M; Serafin A; Sarzi-Puttini P.Feet nailfold capillaroscopy is not useful to detect the typical scleroderma pattern.comment in: Clin Exp Rheumatol. 2013 Mar-Apr;31(2 Suppl 76):189-90; Clinical & Experimental Rheumatology. 30(2 Suppl 71):S116-7, 2012 Mar-Apr.

Pavlov-Dolijanovic S; Damjanov NS; Stojanovic RM; Vujasinovic Stupar NZ; Stanisavljevic DM.Scleroderma pattern of nailfold capillary changes as predictive value for the development of a connective tissue disease: a follow-up study of 3,029 patients with primary Raynaud's phenomenon.Rheumatology International. 32(10):3039-45, 2012 Oct.

Kayser C; Sekiyama JY; Prospero LC; Camargo CZ; Andrade LE.Nailfold capillaroscopy abnormalities as predictors of mortality in patients with systemic sclerosis. Clinical & Experimental Rheumatology. 31(2 Suppl 76):103-8, 2013 Mar-Apr.

Castellvi I; Simeon-Aznar CP; Sarmiento M; Fortuna A; Mayos M; Geli C; Diaz-Torne C; Moya P; De Llobet JM; Casademont J. Association between nailfold capillaroscopy findings and pulmonary function tests in patients with systemic sclerosis. Journal of Rheumatology. 42(2):222-7, 2015 Feb.

Ennis H; Moore T; Murray A; Vail A; Herrick AL.Further confirmation that digital ulcers are associated with the severity of abnormality on nailfold capillaroscopy in patients with systemic sclerosis. Rheumatology. 53(2):376-7, 2014 Feb

Fichel F; Baudot N; Gaitz JP; Trad S; Barbe C; Frances C; Senet P.Systemic sclerosis with normal or nonspecific nailfold capillaroscopy. Dermatology. 228(4):360-7, 2014.

Schlager O; Kiener HP; Stein L; Hofkirchner J; Zehetmayer S; Ristl R; Perkmann T; Smolen JS; Koppensteiner R; Gschwandtner

ME. Associations of nailfold capillary abnormalities and immunological markers in early Raynaud's phenomenon. Scandinavian Journal of Rheumatology. 43(3):226-33, 2014.

Sulli A; Ruaro B; Alessandri E; Pizzorni C; Cimmino MA; Zampogna G; Gallo M; Cutolo M. Correlations between nailfold microangiopathy severity, finger dermal thickness and fingertip blood perfusion in systemic sclerosis patients. Annals of the Rheumatic Diseases. 73(1):247-51, 2014 Jan.

Avouac J; Vallucci M; Smith V; Senet P; Ruiz B; Sulli A; Pizzorni C; Frances C; Chiocchia G; Cutolo M; Allanore Y. Correlations between angiogenic factors and capillaroscopic patterns in systemic sclerosis. Arthritis Research & Therapy. 15(2):R55, 2013.

SYSTEMIC LUPUS ERYTHEMATOSUS

Kuryliszyn-Moskal, A; Ciolkiewicz, M; Klimiuk, P A; Sierakowski, S. Clinical significance of nailfold capillaroscopy in systemic lupus erythematosus: correlation with endothelial cell activation markers and disease activity. Scandinavian Journal of Rheumatology. 38(1):38-45, 2009 Jan-Feb.

SARCOIDOSIS

Santoro F; Sloan SB. Nail dystrophy and bony involvement in chronic sarcoidosis.Comment in: J Am Acad Dermatol. 2010 Jul;63(1):159-60; PMID: 20542178Journal of the American Academy of Dermatology. 60(6):1050-2, 2009 Jun.

DERMATOMYOSITIS

Manfredi A; Sebastiani M; Cassone G; Pipitone N; Giuggioli D; Colaci M; Salvarani C; Ferri C. Nailfold capillaroscopic changes in dermatomyositis and polymyositis. Clinical Rheumatology. 34(2):279-84, 2015 Feb.

ONYCHOMYCOSIS

Onalan O; Adar A; Keles H; Ertugrul G; Ozkan N; Aktas H; Karakaya E.Onychomycosis is associated with subclinical atherosclerosis in patients with diabetes. Vasa. 44(1):59-64, 2015 Jan.

Baran R, Hay RJ, Tosti A *et al* New classification of onychomycosis, Br J Dermatol 119:567–571, 1998.Zaias N Onychomycosis, Dermatol Clin 3: 445–460, 1985

GERIATRIC NAIL FINDINGS

Baran,Robert. The nail in the elderly. [Review] Clinics in Dermatology. 29(1):54-60, 2011 Jan-Feb.

El-Domyati M; Abdel-Wahab H; Abdel-Azim E.

Nail changes and disorders in elderly Egyptians.

Journal of Cosmetic Dermatology. 13(4):269-76, 2014 Dec.

Singh G; Haneef NS; Uday A. Nail changes and disorders among the elderly. [Review] [34 refs]

Indian Journal of Dermatology, Venereology & Leprology. 71(6):386-92, 2005 Nov-Dec.

MISCELLANEOUS NAIL FINDINGS

Yaemsiri S; Hou N; Slining MM; He K. Growth rate of human fingernails and toenails in healthy American young adults.Journal of the European Academy of Dermatology & Venereology. 24(4):420-3, 2010 Apr.

Grzesiak M; Pacan P; Reich A; Szepietowski JC. Onychotillomania in the course of depression: a case report. Acta Dermato-Venereologica. 94(6):745-6, 2014 Nov.

Moghazy D; Sharan C; Nair M; Rackauskas C; Burnette R; Diamond M; Al-Hendy O; Al-Hendy A. Sertoli-Leydig cell tumor with unique nail findings in a post-menopausal woman: a case report and literature review. [Review] Journal of ovarian research. 7:83, 2014.

Allouni A; Yousif A; Akhtar S. Allouni, A; Yousif, A; Akhtar, S. Chronic paronychia in a hairdresser. Occupational Medicine (Oxford). 64(6):468-9, 2014 Sep.

Paparde A; Neringa-Martinsone K; Plakane L; Aivars JI. Nail fold capillary diameter changes in acute systemic hypoxia. Microvascular Research. 93:30-3, 2014 May.

Erdogan AG; Karahacioglu FB; Kavak A. Pterygium unguis in leprosy.International Journal of Dermatology. 52(12):1621-3, 2013 Dec.

Tallon B; Strydom F; Emanuel PO. Nail plate clues to a remote diagnosis. Journal of Cutaneous Pathology. 40(1):2-3, 2013 Jan.

Jha AK; Anand V; Mallik SK; Kumar P..Post Kala azar dermal leishmaniasis (PKDL) presenting with ulcerated chronic paronychia like lesion. Kathmandu University Medical Journal. 10(40):87-90, 2012 Oct-Dec.

Chan HY; Lee DT; Leung EM; Man CW; Lai KM; Leung MW; Wong IK. The effects of a foot and toenail care protocol for older adults. Geriatric Nursing. 33(6):446-53, 2012 Nov-Dec.

Kibby T; Ring DS. Nail injury and diquat exposure: forgotten but not gone. Dermatitis. 23(4):176-8, 2012 Jul-Aug.

Ong GC; Kwah RY; Giam YC .Solitary nail dystrophy in an elderly adult: what lies beneath?. Journal of the American Geriatrics Society. 60(4):789-90, 2012 Apr.

Ferreira O; Baudrier T; Mota A; Duarte AF; Azevedo F. Docetaxel-induced acral erythema and nail changes distributed to photoexposed areas. Cutaneous & Ocular Toxicology. 29(4):296-9, 2010 Dec.

Murynka,Tania. Dermacase. Can you identify this condition? Nail lichen planus. Canadian Family Physician. 55(12):1207-8, 2009 Dec.

Birznieks, Ingvars; Macefield, Vaughan G; Westling, Goran; Johansson, Roland S. Slowly adapting mechanoreceptors in the borders of the human fingernail encode fingertip forces. Journal of Neuroscience. 29(29):9370-9, 2009 Jul 22.

Myers, John B. "Capillary band width", the "nail (band) sign": a clinical marker of microvascular integrity, inflammation, cognition and age. A personal viewpoint and hypothesis. Journal of the Neurological Sciences. 283(1-2):86-90, 2009 Aug 15.

Salem A; Al Mokadem S; Attwa E; Abd El Raoof S; Ebrahim HM; Faheem KT. Nail changes in chronic renal failure patients under haemodialysis. Journal of the European Academy of Dermatology & Venereology. 22(11):1326-31, 2008 Nov.

Chou SL; Chou MY; Kao WF; Yen DH; Huang CI; Lee CH.Cessation of nail growth following Bajiaolian intoxication. Clinical Toxicology: The Official Journal of the American Academy of Clinical Toxicology & European Association of Poisons Centres & Clinical Toxicologists. 46(2):159-63, 2008 Feb.

Carducci M; Calcaterra R; Franco G; Mussi A; Bonifati C; Morrone A.Nail involvement in pemphigus vulgaris. Comment in: Acta Derm Venereol. 2008;88(5):542; PMID: 18779911 Acta Dermato-Venereologica. 88(1):58-60, 2008.

Maeda M; Yamazaki T; Tawada C. Nailfold bleeding of fingers in a mountaineer with severe frostbite. Journal of Dermatology. 34(3):219-20, 2007 Mar.

Gekeler F; Shinoda K; Junger M; Bartz-Schmidt KU; Gelisken F. Familial retinal arterial tortuosity associated with tortuosity in nail bed capillaries. Archives of Ophthalmology. 124(10):1492-4, 2006 Oct.

Pillay I; Lyons D; German MJ; Lawson NS; Pollock HM; Saunders J; Chowdhury S; Moran P; Towler MR. The use of fingernails as a means of assessing bone health: a pilot study. Journal of Women's Health. 14(4):339-44, 2005 May.

Piraccini BM, Iorizzo M, Tosti A. Drug-induced nail abnormalities. Am J Clin Dermatol 4:31-37. 2003

ABOUT THE AUTHOR

Mark E. Williams, MD is the Emeritus Ward K. Ensminger Distinguished Professor of Geriatric Medicine in the Department of Medicine at the University of Virginia. He received his MD degree and Internal Medicine Residency from the University of North Carolina at Chapel Hill. Particularly interested in promoting the health and independence of elderly people, he has authored more than 100 peer-reviewed articles on various aspects of geriatric medicine including pioneering approaches to geriatric assessment, team models of care, uses of advanced communications technology, and the approach to the elderly patient. Currently living in Wilmington, NC he has an active clinical practice spending significant time in outpatient, inpatient, and assisted-living, and nursing home settings. In 1995, Harmony Books, published his book, *The American Geriatrics Society's Complete Guide to Aging & Health*. This book, sometimes called "The Dr. Spock for Older People" is addressed to the general public and aims to empower individuals by allowing them to be better informed and to take a more active role in their own health decisions. McFarland Publishing published his book—*Geriatric Physical Diagnosis: A Guide to Observation and Assessment*—in October 2007. His most recent book is *The Art and Science of Aging Well* published by UNCPress in 2016. He is recognized through peer evaluations in American Health and other surveys as one of the best doctors in America.

Printed in Poland
by Amazon Fulfillment
Poland Sp. z o.o., Wrocław